BRAIN, VISION, MEMORY

D1323396

BRAIN, VISION, MEMORY
Tales in the History of Neuroscience

CHARLES G. GROSS

A BRADFORD BOOK

THE MIT PRESS

CAMBRIDGE, MASSACHUSETTS

LONDON, ENGLAND

First MIT Press paperback edition, 1999

© 1998 Massachusetts Institute of Technology

This book was set in Bembo by Wellington Graphics and was printed and bound in the United States of America.

Library of Congress Cataloging-in-Publication Data

Gross, Charles G.
  Brain, vision, memory : tales in the history of neurosciences /
  Charles G. Gross.
    p.   cm.
  Includes biliographical references and index.
    ISBN 0-262-07186-X (hc : alk. paper), 0-262-57135-8 (pb)
  1. Neurosciences—History.
  QP353.G76   1998
  612.8′09—dc21   97-17168
                                                                        CIP

To Derek

CONTENTS

CONTENTS

I am an experimental neuroscientist specializing in brain mechanisms in vision, and a teacher of neuroscience. This introduction explains what led me temporarily to put aside my experiments and neglect my students to write the five tales on the history of neuroscience.

The first essay began in 1960. I had just completed the experimental work for my Ph.D. thesis, "Some Alterations in Behavior after Frontal Lesions in Monkeys," at Cambridge University and sat down to write the requisite review of the literature. Six months later I had reached Galen and the second century. At that point, my advisor, Larry Weiskrantz, suggested that, actually, it might be better if I got on with the write-up of my experiments, even though, as I explained to him, Galen had carried out experiments on frontal lobe damage in piglets. So I never included this historical survey in my thesis, and ultimately its review of previous work began with studies in the 1930s.

I did show my "up to Galen" manuscript to Joseph Needham. He wrote me an encouraging note, resplendent with Chinese characters, comparing Greek pneuma with Chinese chi. After graduate school I went to the Massachusetts Institute of Technology as a postdoctoral fellow to work with Hans-Lukas Teuber, the charismatic founder of the Department of Psychology, now the Department of Brain and Cognitive Sciences (Gross, 1994a). I showed him my history manuscript and proposed to continue working on it on the side. Teuber was deeply knowledgeable about the history of biology, almost as deeply as he pretended to be; however, he assured me that I had no time "on the side" and should save history for my retirement days.

Despite this advice, when I began to teach what became my perennial undergraduate course on physiological psychology (later renamed cognitive neuroscience), first at Harvard and then at Princeton, I increasingly inserted historical interludes on Vesalius, Willis, and Gall, and other "high points in man's understanding of his brain." When some of the premedical students in the course started getting restless at the length of these interludes, I began occasionally teaching a separate course entitled "Ideas on Brain Function from Antiquity to the Twentieth Century."

After the (perceived) success, described below, of my paper on the hippocampus minor, I reached into my "up to Galen" draft and my history of neuroscience lecture notes and began revising and updating them for publication. So when I was asked a few years ago to write an article on visual cortex for the multivolume handbook *Cerebral Cortex* I seized the opportunity to achieve my thwarted ambition to write a historical introduction starting at the beginning. I began with the first written mention of the brain from the pyramid age, went on to investigations and theories of brain function among Greek physician-philosopher-scientists, and continued through the coma of European science between Galen and the Renaissance. At that point in the article, for obvious practical reasons (my word limit and, certainly, my time were not infinite), I began to narrow my subject, first to the cerebral cortex and then, by the end of the article, to striate cortex. Chapter 1, "From Imhotep to Hubel and Wiesel: The Story of Visual Cortex" is a combination of that article (Gross, 1997c) and one I wrote entitled "Aristotle and the Brain" for the *Neuroscientist* (Gross, 1995).

The second essay was inspired by a visit to an exhibit of Leonardo's anatomical drawings at the Metropolitan Museum of Art in New York. The rooms were dimly lit and the hushed crowd slowly and reverentially shifted from drawing to drawing of bones, muscles, and viscera, all borrowed from the

Queen's collection at Windsor Castle. No pamphlets were available nor were there explanations on the walls, not even labels or dates of the drawings. What were we looking at? The drawings of the superficial musculature seemed accurate enough and certainly beautiful. But the viscera often seemed rather strange, the organs not looking quite right or in the correct places. Of course, I had previously seen his two drawings of brain ventricles, one a purely medieval three circles in the head and the other a realistic, but not quite human ventricular system. I became intrigued as to what Leonardo was illustrating in these famous drawings: the body observed? the body remembered? the body read about? the body rumored? the human body, or animals in human form? Was he illustrating medieval theory, as in the drawing of circular ventricles? Or was he drawing from his own dissection, as in the later ventricular drawing? Hence, eventually, the article on Leonardo's anatomy. Although it is restricted to a detailed discussion of only a few of Leonardo's neuroanatomical drawings, I think my comments are applicable to his other biological work. Chapter 2, "Leonardo da Vinci on the Eye and Brain," was first published in the *Neuroscientist* (Gross, 1997b).

The third essay derived from the question of whether there can be a theoretical biology or a theoretical biologist. Certainly I see no sign yet of anyone who made significant and lasting theoretical contributions while remaining only a theorist. All the great theoretical work was done by individuals buried up to their necks if not their eyebrows with empirical data all their busy lives, such as Darwin, Mendel, Bernard, Sherrington, and even Freud. In contrast, those individuals who were only theorists and did little empirical slogging, such as Lotka, Reshevsky, and D'arcy Thompson, have disappeared except as antiquarian curios.

Was Emmanuel Swedenborg, the eighteenth-century Swedish mystic, an exception? Solely on the basis of reading the literature of the day, he proposed theories of the functions of the cerebral cortex, of the organization of motor cortex, and of the functions of the pituitary gland that were at least 200 years ahead of everyone else. On the other hand, perhaps he was no exception since, although he often got it right, he never had any impact on biology. Indeed, his work was published and republished in many volumes, but his ideas on the brain continued to go unnoticed until after those that were actually correct were rediscovered independently. Chapter 3, "Emanual Swedenborg: A Neuroscientist Before His Time," first published in the *Neuroscientist,* tells his story (Gross, 1997a).

The fourth essay originated when my wife, Greta Berman, bought me a copy of Desmond and Moore's biography of Darwin soon after it appeared. She had been attracted by a very enthusiastic blurb on the back cover written by a friend of ours. At first I was skeptical, as the book had been rather negatively reviewed in the *New York Times Book Review* by my old history of science teacher, I. B. Cohen. But as soon as I began to read, I realized what an absolutely splendid book it was, a truly exciting page turner placing Darwin in his social, economic, and scientific world.

Right in the middle of the book I encountered several references to a lobe of the brain called the hippocampus minor. I do sometimes come across names of unfamiliar brain structures, but never a whole lobe, particularly one that was supposed to be unique to humans. As I looked into more accounts of Victorian biology and the battles over evolution, I realized that although the hippocampus minor was repeatedly mentioned by historians of evolution, it was clear that none of them had any idea of what or where it was. Apparently they had never read or even looked at the pictures in the many articles about the hippocampus minor in midnineteenth-century scientific and popular journals. Furthermore, I could find no mention of such a structure in any of my neuroanatomy textbooks (until later when I looked at outdated ones). When I called several of my friends around the country who were among the leading students of the anatomy and physiology of the hippocampus, they too had never heard of the hippocampus minor. Clearly, there was or should have been a ready audience for a paper on this mysterious structure. Hence I researched and wrote "The Hippocampus Minor and Man's Place in Nature: A Case Study in the Social Construction of Neuroanatomy," a version of which constitutes chapter 4. It tells what the hippocampus minor is, why it was so important in the controversies that swirled around Darwin, and why it is now so completely forgotten.

I could not resist publishing it in a journal called *Hippocampus,* which is devoted to studies on the anatomy, physiology, and functions of that structure (Gross, 1993a). I liked my article so much that I published a shorter version entitled "Huxley versus Owen: The Hippocampus Minor and Evolution" in the less specialized, more widely read journal, *Trends in Neuroscience* (Gross, 1993b). Both versions were well received. Indeed, I received more letters of praise for them than I had in response to the over 200 straight science papers I had previously written. I was so reinforced by this reception, as we used to say in B. F. Skinner's heyday, that over the next few years I submitted for publication several other history of neuroscience articles: versions of them make up the rest of this book.

The fifth essay arose when I was asked to organize a conference on object recognition and the temporal lobes at the Massachusetts Institute of Technology in honor of Hans-Lukas Teuber in 1993. After the conference, Pat Goldman-Rakic, the editor of the journal *Cerebral Cortex,* asked me to edit a special issue based on the meeting. I decided to add a history article of my own to introduce the issue. The article, entitled "How Inferior Temporal Cortex Became a Visual Area," traced how the visual functions of the temporal cortex were discovered (Gross, 1994b). My colleagues and I had been the first to record from neurons in the temporal cortex (we did so at MIT, under Teuber's sponsorship), so I made the account of this work at the end of the article very personal and autobiographical. Chapter 5, "Beyond the Striate Cortex: How Large Portions of the Temporal and Parietal Cortex Became Visual Areas," is derived in part from that article. I expanded its scope to include not only the temporal lobe but also how the parietal lobe became a visual area. Both developments followed from nineteenth-century observations on the effect of temporal and parietal lesions in monkeys that were forgotten and had to be subsequently rediscovered.

Greta Berman, Michael Graziano, and Hillary Rodman read all the essays at least once and gave many helpful comments and much encouragement.

Several of the essays were improved by the detailed comments of David Czuchlewski, George Krauthamer, Larry Squire, Derek Gross, Phil Johnson-Laird, Mort Mishkin, Maz Fallah, and Robert Young. Maggie Berkowitz and John Cooper were particularly helpful with the classical material. George Krauthamer was kind enough to dissect the hippocampus minor of a human and several species of primates for my benefit, as well as translate from the German, Dutch, and French. Steve Waxman, founding editor of the *Neuroscientist,* encouraged the entire project by publishing two of the essays and signing me up for lots more in the future. Linda Chamberlin of the Princeton University Library was tireless in getting me old books and journals from everywhere. Mairi Benson, librarian of the Sherrington Collection in the History of Neuroscience in the Physiological Laboratories, Oxford University, was also very helpful, as was the Wellcome Institute Library in London. I thank Michael Rutter and Katherine Arnoldi, editors at The MIT Press, for their assistance and tolerance, Sarah Jeffries for copy editing the manuscript, and Shalani Alisharan for proofreading and making the index.

Some support came from a McDonnell-Pew Fellowship in Cognitive Neuroscience at Oxford University, and the preparation of the accounts of modern visual neuroscience was helped by National Eye Institute grant EY 11347-26. Finally, and particularly crucial for every phase of the entire enterprise was the unstinting help of Nina Rebmann and Maida Rosengarten.

BRAIN, VISION, MEMORY

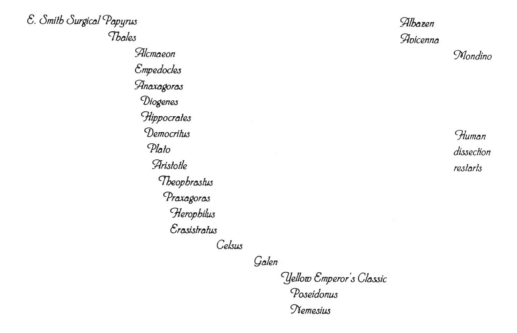

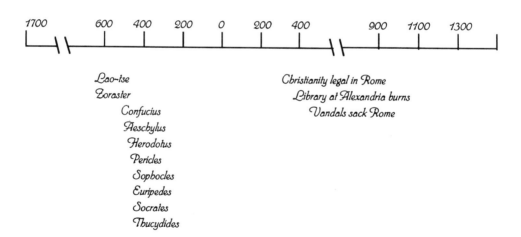

The upper time line shows when each of the major Pre-Renaissance figures discussed in this book flourished. The lower one indicates some contemporaneous figures and events.

Leonardo.......   Owen.................
  Vesalius...   Darwin.............
    Piccolomini................... Spencer............
      Descartes..   Broca........
      Bartholin......   Huxley.........
      Willis.......   Jackson...........
       Malpighi.......   Hitsig............
        Ruysch................. Fritsch.................
         Newton............ Munk.............
          Pourfour du Petit   James...........
           Swedenborg........ Ferrier...............
            Linnaeus.......   Flechsig.............
             Haller........... Loeb............
              Lamarck............ Beck...............
               Gennari...   Brodman..
               Gall............... Campbell.........
                Bell............... E. Smith.......
                 Spurzheim..   Economo....
                  Tiedemann........ Holmes...............
                   Panizza............. Inouye.................
                    Flourens.......... Adrian................
                     Müller.......   Lashley.........

    1500   1600   1700   1800   1900

Copernicus, "De Revolutionibus..."
    Harvey, "On the Movement of the Heart..."
    Galileo, "Dialogues on Two New Sciences"
        Locke, "Essay Concerning Human Understanding"
        Berkeley, "New Theory of Vision"
            Galvani, frog experiments
                Wöhler synthesizes urea
                Babbage conceives computer
                Schleiden / Schwann, cell theory
                Helmholtz, conduction speed
                Sechenov, "Reflexes..."
                Bernard, le milieu interieur
                Cajal, neuron theory

The upper time line shows the birth (initial letter) and death (final dot) of the major Post-Renaissance figures discussed in this book. The lower gives the year of major events relevant to the development of modern neuroscience.

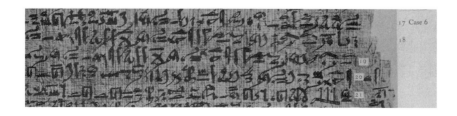

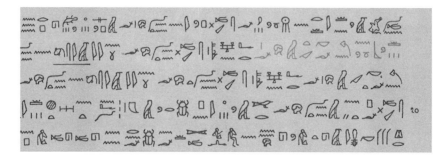

Figure 1.1 A portion of the Edwin Smith surgical papyrus, case six, concerning a skull fracture that exposed the cortex (Breasted, 1930). Upper, the actual papyrus, written in a hieratic script. Lower, the hieroglyphic transliteration. The word for brain is underlined. Writing is left to right in both figures. (Princeton University Library)

From Imhotep to Hubel and Wiesel:
The Story of Visual Cortex

This chapter traces the origins of our current ideas about visual cortex. I begin in the thirtieth century BCE with the earliest description of the cerebral cortex. In the second part I consider the views of Greek philosopher-scientists on the functions of the brain. The third part concerns the long period in which there were virtually no advances in Europe in understanding the brain or any other aspect of the natural world. In the fourth part I describe how even after brain research was again well under way, the cerebral cortex tended to be ignored. The fifth section considers the beginning of the modern study of the cerebral cortex and the localization therein of psychological functions. Our focus narrows in the sixth section, and I address how a specifically visual area of the cortex was delineated. The chapter ends with the award of the Nobel prize to David Hubel and Thorsten Wiesel in 1981 for their discoveries about visual cortex.

Ancient Egyptian Surgery and Medicine

The First Written Mention of the Brain

The first written reference to the cortex, indeed to any part of the brain, occurs in the Edwin Smith surgical papyrus (figure 1.1). Although written about

1700 BCE, this papyrus is a copy of a much older surgical treatise dating back to the pyramid age of the Old Kingdom (about thirtieth century BCE). The papyrus was bought in 1862 by an American Egyptologist, Edwin Smith, from a local in Luxor, probably one of the "hereditary" tomb robbers who inhabit a nearby village. It eventually found its way to the great American Egyptologist James H. Breasted.[1]

The publication of Breasted's translation in 1930 made an enormous impact on medical historians and Egyptologists.[2] Previously, Egyptian medicine had been thought to be a jumble of incantations, amulets, and superstitions. Rational medicine was supposed to begin only with the Greeks. Yet, the Edwin Smith papyrus is clear evidence of a scientific observer attempting to understand the human body and to treat, rationally, its injury.

The papyrus consists of a coolly empirical description of forty-eight cases, starting from the head and working down to the shoulders, where the copyist stops in midsentence. For each case, the author systematically describes the examination, diagnosis, and feasibility of treatment. Each diagnosis comes to one of three conclusions: that the patient should be told that it is "an ailment that I will treat," "an ailment that I will try to treat," or "an ailment that I will not treat."

The word for brain first comes up in case six, a person with a skull fracture:

> (*Title*) Instructions concerning a gaping wound in his head, penetrating to the bone, smashing his skull, (and) rending open the brain of his skull.
>
> (*Examination*) If thou examinest a man having a gaping wound in his head, penetrating to the bone, smashing his skull, and rending open the brain of his skull, thou shouldst palpate his wound. Shouldst thou find that smash which is in his skull [like] those corrugations which form in molten copper, (and) something therein throbbing (and) fluttering under thy fingers, like the weak place of an infant's crown before it becomes whole . . . (and) he

[the patient] discharges blood from both his nostrils, (and) he suffers
with stiffness in his neck.
(Diagnosis) [you say] an ailment not to be treated.[3]

And indeed, the "corrugations" that form in molten copper during the smelting
process such as that of early Egypt really do look like cerebral cortex.

In several cases, the author notes the relation of the laterality of the injury
to the laterality of the symptom. For example, in case five, the patient "walks
shuffling with his sole on the side of him having that injury which is in his
skull." (Presumably, a contracoup injury; that is, a blow to one side of the head
that causes the brain to shift within the cranium and make impact on the inside
of the contralateral skull, thereby causing damage contralateral to the site of the
blow.)

The author was clearly aware that the site of injury determines the locus
and nature of the symptoms. Thus, in case thirty-one, "It is a dislocation of a
vertebra of the neck extending to this backbone which causes him to be
unconscious of his two arms and legs." Elsewhere, the author mentions the
meninges and the cerebrospinal fluid, and describes aphasia ("he speaks not to
thee") and seizures ("he shudders exceedingly").

Although the document is startling in its rationality and empiricism and
in the virtual absence of superstition and magic, Breasted did tend to overin-
terpret the papyrus; he wrote, for example, "this recognition of the localization
of function in the brain . . . shows an astonishing early discernment which has
been more fully developed by modern surgeons only within the present generations."[4] Perhaps Breasted's greatest flight of fancy was the suggestion that
the papyrus was written by Imhotep, a famous physician who flourished about
the time the original of the papyrus was written. There is absolutely no evidence
that he wrote it, however; in fact, he is very unlikely to have done so, since
the papyrus deals largely with battle wounds, and in the rigidly hierarchical
world of Egyptian medicine, Imhotep was certainly not a battlefield surgeon.

He certainly was, however, an interesting figure in his own right.[5] He
was the grand vizier of the third dynasty Pharaoh Zoser (2700–2650 BCE). A

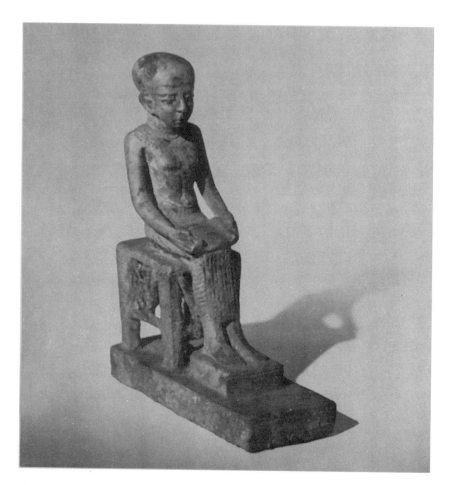

Figure 1.2 A statuette of Imhotep as a demigod, a person of human origin who after his death was viewed as superhuman and worshipped. He achieved this status within 100 years of his death. As a demigod, Imhotep was typically represented with an open scroll on his lap. Statuettes like this one, from the Civica Raccolta Egizia in Milan, must have been common, as there are, for example, forty-eight in the Wellcome Historical Medical Museum, twenty-one in the Cairo Museum, about fifty in the Louvre, and ten in the Hermitage (Hurray, 1928).

contemporary inscription describes him as "chancellor of the king of Lower Egypt, the first after the King of Upper Egypt, administrator of the great palace, hereditary noble, high priest of Heliopolis, the builder, the sculptor." He is credited with designing the step pyramid of Sakkara, which was the tomb of Zoser, the first pyramid, and the first example of large-scale dressed stone architecture. He was also a priest, astrologer, and magician. Yet his fame as a physician seems to have impressed his contemporaries and later generations most of all. Miniature statues of him were used as amulets to ward off disease (figure 1.2), and eventually, he was deified as the Egyptian god of medicine (figure 1.3), an unusual honor even for a successful physician.[6, 7]

The Legacy of Egyptian Medicine

The period of the Middle Kingdom (starting about 2000 BCE) saw a gradual decline in the artistic, architectural, and intellectual creativity and vibrancy that characterized the earlier dynasties. The society became more rigid and hierarchical, intellectual life more dominated by priests, sculptures were largely copies of earlier works, and buildings more gigantic and grandiose. The rational and empirical spirit of medical practice that suffuses the Edwin Smith papyrus largely gave way to mysticism, religion, and elaborate speculations on the next world.[8] Yet, the fame of ancient Egyptian medicine lived on, in the *Odyssey,* in the Old Testament, among the presocratic physicians, in Galen, in the Cabala, and today, in any New Age boutique or "health food" store.

It is important to view the correlations between brain injury and symptom in the Smith papyrus in the context of ancient Egyptian medical theory and practice. We know that the Egyptians thought that the heart was the most important organ in the body, the seat of the mind, and the center of intellectual activities. This is clear from their philosophical and religious writings, and emphasized by their practice of mummification. Both Herodotus's descriptions[9] of the process of embalming and later examination of mummies show the contrast between the importance of the heart and brain in Egyptian thought. The first step in mummification was to scoop out the brain through the nostrils

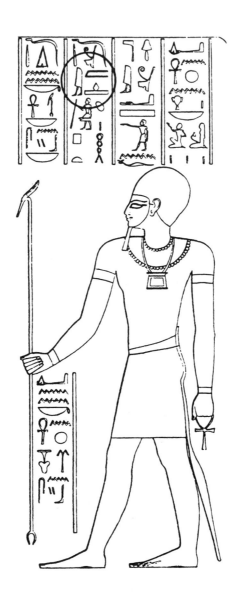

with an iron bar. In contrast, the heart (and most other internal organs) was either elaborately wrapped and replaced in the body or carefully stored in canopic jars near the body. As indicated in the *Book of the Dead,* ancient Egyptians considered it essential that the body be preserved and all the important organs be retained so that in the afterlife the body would be in a suitable condition for resurrection when the soul returned to it. Dead Pharaohs were prepared for their next life with everything but a brain.

The idea of the heart as the sensory and intellectual center of the body seems to have been universal, as it occurs also in other ancient civilizations such as Mesopotamia, Babylonia, and India.[10, 11] It is reported to be common among preliterature cultures,[12] as well, as illustrated by the oft-quoted remark of a Pueblo chief to C.G. Jung,[13] "I know you white men think with the brain. That accounts for your shortcomings. We red men think with the heart." Ancient Chinese medicine held rather more complicated views than the relatively simple heart-centered ones, but it also seems to have largely ignored the brain.[14] In fact, the role of the brain in perception and cognition does not appear to enter Chinese thought until the Jesuit Matteo Ricci's treatise (1595, in Chinese) on the art of memory, which he wrote as part of his campaign to convert the scholar class.[15]

As we will see, the view that the heart was the seat of sensation and thought was even held by the greatest of all savants, Aristotle. It persisted for over a millennium, together with the more prevalent theory that the brain, not the heart, was crucial for these functions.

Figure 1.3 Imhotep as the Egyptian god of medicine. The earliest known divine representation of Imhoptep dates from about 525 BCE, about twenty-five centuries his death. This painting is from the temple of Ptah at Karnak. Typical for a god, he wears a ceremonial beard and carries a scepter in his right hand and an ankh in his left, and a lion's tail is attached to his belt. The hieroglyphs representing an abbreviated version of his name are circled. The most famous temple devoted to Imhotep was at Memphis, and became a hospital and school of medicine and magic. By Ptolemaic times Imhotep was assimilated into the Greek god of medicine, Asclepias (Hurray, 1928).

GREEK PHILOSOPHER-SCIENTISTS AND
THE BEGINNING OF BRAIN SCIENCE

The approach to head injury of the Edwin Smith surgical papyrus stands out as a rock of empiricism in the sea of mysticism and superstition in which biological and medical writings in the Near East swam for about the next twenty-four centuries. Even so, one could hardly call the papyrus scientific. Science is not just craft or knowledge. Medical science is not just description of symptoms or treatment, and it is not just the absence of superstition or magic. Rather, science, or perhaps we should say formal, self-conscious science, is the assumption that the world can be understood by human reason, a mechanism that works in some consistent way with a regularity governed by a limited set of rules. In this scientific world view, the universe is not the playground of gods and ghosts acting in a capricious fashion, moved by passion and whim. Science is public: it demands rational, critical debate; it involves observation, description, and measurement; it carries the assumption that underlying principles or laws are potentially accessible by these methods.

This idea of formal science begins, at least in the West, with a group of Greek thinkers known as presocratic philosophers.[16] They used the term *physiologia* to describe themselves, which is perhaps best translated as "natural philosophers," rather than physiologists, physicists, or just philosophers.

Miletus, Cradle of Science

The earliest presocratics came from Miletus, one of a set of Greek city-states in Ionia, located on the west shore of modern Turkey (figure 1.4). What was special about this time and place that made it the cradle of science? The Ionians were a Greek people deriving from Crete. They were pioneers living in a new land and creating a new set of political institutions. The Bronze Age was becoming the Iron Age, enabling the cheap production of tools and weapons, and thus these city-states could maintain themselves, at least for a while, in the face of the empires to their East. By the sixth century BCE, Miletus was a great

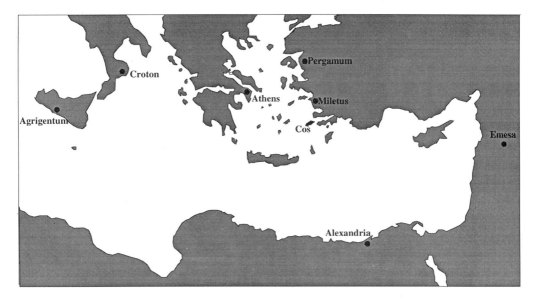

Figure 1.4   Some of the important centers of classical medicine and biology.

port city that had established trading colonies throughout the Mediterranean and Black seas. It was a meeting of the sea lanes of Greek, Phoenician, and Egyptian traders and the overland caravans from the East as far as India and China. Its wealth derived both from its merchant ships and from local industries such as textiles and pottery. With its rich ferment of races, cultures, and ideas, Miletus was an interface between East and West.

At about this time, the rule of the landed aristocracy was breaking up and power was going to the merchant classes. They had the wealth to support speculation on the nature of the universe, and they had the desire for new techniques, particularly in math and astronomy. In addition, the development of alphabetic writing broke the monopoly held by the class of scribe-priests that characterized the cuneiform and hieroglyphic civilizations. The Ionian philosophers were neither prophets nor priests, but usually inventors, engineers, traders, or politicians, and often several of these at once. Slavery was not yet so pervasive that the ruling classes regarded manual labor with contempt.

Finally, in these new city-states there was debate about the nature of society and about the best form of government. These freedoms to question the nature of social institutions seem to have been part of the spirit of inquiry into the physical and biological world. All this ferment bubbled up into the beginning of the systematic examination of the universe that we call science.

Thales (ca. 583) was the first of the presocratic philosophers and thus is traditionally named the first (Western) scientist. He visited Egypt, returned with a number of geometric facts, and applied them to practical problems such as measuring the height of a building and the distance of a ship at sea. He seems to have been the first to conceive of the value of a general proposition or theorem in geometry. He is credited with such proofs as that the base angles of an isosceles triangle are equal and a circle is bisected by its diameter.[17]

Thales is most famous, however, for his idea that water was the basic and original substance. He thought that the earth was a flat disk floating on water, that water was all around the world, and that the heavenly bodies were water vapor. What is new or scientific about this? After all, the Egyptians, the Babylonians, and indeed all peoples have cosmologies about how things began, and water cosmologies are particularly common. For example, in one Babylonian legend[18] the creator is Marduk and "All the lands were sea . . . Marduk bound a rush mat upon the face of the waters, he made dirt and piled it on the rush mat." Thales's cosmology was fundamentally different from the Babylonian and other prescientific ones for two reasons. First, he left gods such as Marduk out of his scheme. Second, he sought a common element underlying all phenomena.

Alcmaeon of Croton, the First Neuroscientist

By the middle of the fifth century BCE there were three major centers of Greek medical science: Croton, in what is now southern Italy, Agrigentum on the south coast of modern Sicily, and Cos, an island off modern Turkey. The oldest was in Croton, and its most famous member was Alcmaeon.

Alcmaeon (ca. 450) was the first writer to champion the brain as the site of sensation and cognition.[19] He also seems to have been the first practitioner of anatomic dissection as a tool of intellectual inquiry. His most detailed dissections and theories were on the senses, particularly vision. Alcmaeon described the optic nerves and noted that they came together "behind the forehead" (which is why, he opined, the eyes move together) and suggested that they were "light-bearing paths" to the brain. He removed and dissected the eye and observed that it contained water. Observations of what are now called phosphenes occurring after a blow to the eye led him to conclude that the eye also contained light (fire) and that this light was necessary for vision. This became the basis of theories of vision that persisted beyond the Renaissance. Indeed, Alcmaeon's idea of light in the eye was only disproved in the middle of the eighteenth century.[20]

Among the other presocratic philosopher-scientists who adopted and expanded on Alcmaeon's view of the functions of the brain were Democritus, Anaxagoras, and Diogenes[21] (all ca. 425). Democritus developed a version that became especially influential because of its impact on Plato. Specifically, Democritus taught that everything in the universe is made up of atoms of different sizes and shapes. The psyche (soul, mind, vital principle) is made up of the lightest, most spherical, and fastest-moving atoms. Although the psychic atoms are dispersed among other atoms throughout the body, they are especially numerous in the brain. Slightly cruder atoms are concentrated in the heart, making it the center of emotion, and still cruder ones are located in the liver, which consequently is the seat of lust and appetite. As discussed in the next section, this trichotomy developed into Plato's hierarchy of the parts of the soul. Then, much later, in Galen's medical theorizing, these three parts became the three pneumas of humoral physiology that dominated medical thought for centuries.[22]

Alcmaeon's view of the hegemony of the brain was not universal among the presocratic philosopher-scientists. For example, Empedocles (ca. 445), the leading member of the medical center at Agrigentum, the second great center of Greek medicine, taught that the blood was the medium of thought, and the degree of intelligence depended on the composition of the blood.[23] Thus, for him, the heart was the central organ of intellect and the seat of mental disorder, as it had been among Near Eastern civilizations.

The Hippocratic Doctors

The third great center for the teaching and practice of medicine in the fifth century BCE was the island of Cos, and its most famous member was Hippocrates (ca. 425). The first large body of Western scientific writings that have survived is the Hippocratic corpus. Although there is no question that Hippocrates was a real historical figure, it is not clear which of the works called Hippocratic he actually wrote. The corpus consists of over sixty treatises that vary enormously in style and technical level, and that were not written by one author or even in one period. It may have been the remaining part of the medical library at Cos or, alternatively, it may have been assembled some time later in Alexandria.[24]

Unlike Alcmaeon and the Croton School, the Hippocratic doctors did not practice dissection and their knowledge of anatomy was slight. Like presocratic thinkers in general, however, they rejected supernatural causes of disease and sought natural explanations through observation and extended case studies. Such detailed studies of disease processes were rare until after the Renaissance, and even then they tended to be advertisements for the skill of the physician rather than empirical studies.

The Hippocratic work of greatest relevance to brain function is the famed essay "On the Sacred Disease," that is, epilepsy. Probably designed as a lecture for laymen, it opens with an homage to reason and a rejection of superstition[25]:

> I do not believe that the "Sacred Disease" is any more divine or sacred than any other disease, but, on the contrary, has specific characteristics and a definite cause. . .
>
> It is my opinion that those who first called this disease "sacred" were the sort of people we now call witch-doctors, faith-healers, quacks, and charlatans. These are exactly the people who pretend to be very pious and to be particularly wise. By invoking a divine element they were able to screen their own failure to give suitable treatment and so called this a "sacred" malady to conceal their ignorance of its nature.

The author has no doubt that the brain is the seat of this disease. As to the general functions of the brain, he is equally clear:

It ought to be generally known that the source of our pleasure, merriment, laughter, and amusement, as of our grief, pain, anxiety, and tears, is none other than the brain. It is specially the organ which enables us to think, see, and hear, and to distinguish the ugly and the beautiful, the bad and the good, pleasant and unpleasant . . . It is the brain too which is the seat of madness and delirium, of the fears and frights which assail us, often by night, but sometimes even by day; it is there where lies the cause of insomnia and sleep-walking, of thoughts that will not come, forgotten duties, and eccentricities.

Furthermore, he states that neither the diaphragm nor the heart has any mental functions, as some claimed: "Neither of these organs takes any part in mental operations, which are completely undertaken by the brain."

What then is the cause of epilepsy, the so-called sacred disease? It attacks only the phlegmatic, those with an excess of phlegm or mucus.

Should . . . [the] . . . routes for the passage of phlegm from the brain be blocked, the discharge enters the blood-vessels . . . this causes aphonia, choking, foaming at the mouth, clenching of the teeth and convulsive movements of the hands; the eyes are fixed, the patient becomes unconscious and, in some cases, passes a stool . . . All these symptoms are produced when cold phlegm is discharged into the blood which is warm, so chilling the blood and obstructing its flow.

These extracts typify Hippocratic medicine: absence of superstition, accurate clinical description, ignorance of anatomy, and physiology that is largely a mixture of false analogy, speculation, and humoral theory. Perhaps the entire history of medicine can be viewed as the narrowing of the gap between the medical empiricism characteristic of the School of Cos and the knowledge of structure and mechanism sought by the School of Croton.

Finally, it should be noted that the Hippocratic oath not only had no connection with the Hippocratic School but is quite deviant from mainstream Greek medical and social practice in several ways.[26] In its original form it forbids both suicide and abortion, but, in fact, neither was censured or illegal in Hippocratic times, or more generally, in classical Greece and Rome. The oath also forbids surgery. Although surgical intervention was not common, it was definitely carried out by Hippocratic doctors to drain pus, set fractures, and reduce dislocations. Finally, Hippocratic doctors, like most others before and after, taught for a fee, despite the oath's injunctions against such practices. The so-called Hippocratic oath seems to have derived from a later secret neopythagorean sect that was antisuicide, antiabortion, and antisurgery. It may then have become popular with the rise of Christianity, since the Church was opposed to suicide and abortion, and with the separation of medicine from the "lower craft" of surgery.

Plato: Antiscientist

Plato (427–347 BCE) was unsympathetic to what we and the presocratics meant by science: the empirical investigation of the universe. Indeed, because of the beauty and subtlety of his dialogues, and his towering reputation outside of science, particularly in ethics and politics, Plato can be considered one of the most important ideological opponents of natural science of all time. Furthermore, he dominated European philosophy until about the twelfth century, when Aristotle began to filter into Europe through Muslim civilization. As we will see later, Aristotle, unlike Plato, was very heavily involved in and enthusiastic about scientific investigation.

Plato was born in Athens at a time when that city was the center of the Greek intellectual world. He came from an aristocratic background and was Socrates's most famous student. After Socrates was executed for subversion by the Athenian democracy, Plato left Athens and traveled widely for about a dozen years. He then returned to Athens at the age of forty and founded a school, the Academy, where he taught primarily politics and ethics for another four decades until his death.

Whereas the presocratic philosophers sought laws independent of the supernatural, Plato made "natural laws subordinate to the authority of divine principle," as Plutarch put it. Furthermore, whereas, most of the earlier natural philosophers stressed observation over reason alone, Plato took the opposite view[27]:

> [The universe is] to be apprehended by reason and intelligence, but not by sight (*Republic,* 529).

> . . . If we are to know anything absolutely we must be free from the body and behold actual realities with the eye of the soul alone (*Phaedo,* 66).

In the *Republic* (529–30) Plato ridicules the observational approach of the astronomer:

> The starry heavens . . . are to be apprehended by reason and intelligence, but not by sight . . . a true astronomer will never imagine that the proportions of night, day or both to the month, or of the month to the year . . . and any other things that are material and visible can also be external and subject to no deviation—that would be absurd; and it is equally absurd to take so much pains in establishing their exact truth.

He is similarly opposed to the experimental acoustics of the Pythagoreans, as in this exchange between Glaucon and Socrates (*Rep.,* 531):

> *Socrates:* The teachers of harmony compare the sounds and consonances which are heard only, and their labor, like that of the astronomers is in vain.

Glaucon: Yes, by heaven! And it is as good as a play to hear them talking about their condensed notes, as they call them; they put their ears close alongside of the strings like persons catching a sound from their neighbor's wall—one set of them declaring that they distinguish an intermediate note and have found the least interval which should be the unit of measurement; the others insisting that the two sounds have passed into the same—either party setting their ears before their understanding.

Socrates: You mean those gentlemen who tease and torture the strings and rack them on the pegs of the instrument . . . they too are in error, like the astronomers; they investigate the num- bers of the harmonies which are heard, but they never attain to problems.

Plato's rejection of the possibility of a biology of behavior is similarly total, as in this ridicule of Anaxagoras by the now condemned Socrates in *Phaedo* (97–99):

Then I heard someone reading, as he said, from a book of Anaxagoras, that mind was the disposer and cause of all . . . What expectations I had formed, and how grievously was I disappointed! As I proceeded, I found my philosopher altogether forsaking mind or any other principle of order, but having recourse to air, and ether, water, and other eccentricities. I might compare him to a person who began by maintaining generally that mind is the cause of the actions of Socrates, but who, when he endeavored to explain the causes of my several actions in detail, went on to show that I sit here because my body is made up of bones and muscles; and the bones, he would say, are hard and have joints which divide them, and the muscles are elastic, and they cover the bones, which have also a covering or environment of flesh and skin which contains them; and as the bones are lifted at their joints by the contraction or relaxation of the muscles, I am able to bend my limbs, and this is why I am sitting here in a curved posture—that is what he would say; and he would have a similar explanation of my talking to you, which he would attribute to sound, and air, and hearing and he would assign ten thousand other causes of the same sort, forgetting to mention the true cause, which is, that the Athenians have thought fit to condemn me, and accordingly I have thought it better and more right to remain here and undergo my sentence; . . . to say that I do as I do because of my muscles and bones and that this is the way in which mind acts, and not from the choice of the best, is a very careless and idle mode of speaking.

Whereas Anaxagoras and the other presocratics were searching for a mechanistic cause of behavior, Plato's conception of cause was a teleological one, or, perhaps it might be better called an ethical one.

Plato did more than satirize the methods and goals of the presocratics. He offered an alternative program. He taught that things we see are only superficial appearances, shadows in a cave, and hardly worth serious consideration. Corresponding to each kind of object are Ideas or Forms that are both the origin and the cause of objects that we see. For example, there are various cups in the sensory world, all of which are different, imperfect, and transient. In contrast, the Idea or Form of a cup is perfect and eternal—the archetype of all cups past, present, and future. The goal of the philosopher is to understand these ideas and especially the higher ones such as Virtue, or the highest of all, the Idea of God. The philosopher must escape the tyranny of sensory experience and empirical knowledge and climb out of the cave in order to reach the higher realities of true knowledge (*Rep.*, VII).

Plato's views on the brain were set out in most detail in the *Timaeus* (pp. 69–71), his cosmological essay that was extraordinarily influential in the Middle Ages. The soul, which is prior to the body, is divine and comes from the soul of the universe. It is divided into three parts, following Democritus's three levels of atoms. Reason or intellect is the highest and immortal part and lies in the brain, which controls the rest of the body. In his words "It is the divinest part of us and lords over all the rest," The higher division of the mortal soul lies in the heart. To avoid it polluting the divine soul a neck was built between the two. Appetite, the lowest division, was placed in the liver, "tethered like a beast . . . as far as possible from the seat of counsel" in the head. In the *Republic* (435–442) the three parts of the soul are compared with the three classes of Plato's Utopia. Just as the divine soul or reason must be kept separate from base sensation and appetite, so must rulers be protected from contamination by the masses.

The *Timaeus* did convey presocratic and Hippocratic ideas about the brain, body and, more generally, the universe to the Middle Ages It was particularly successful in spreading Plato's teleology and his rejection of sensation and observation in favor of reason. Thus, modern historians of science have referred to its role in the history of science as "nefarious," "essentially evil," and "an aberration."[28]

Aristotle on Brain and Heart

Aristotle's name is invariably linked to philosophy; indeed, for centuries he was known as "The Philosopher." He was also the leading biologist of classical antiquity and one of the greatest biologists of all times.[29] He is usually considered the founder of comparative anatomy, the first embryologist, the first taxonomist, the first evolutionist, the first biogeographer, and the first systematic student of animal behavior. Not only was he important to the development of biology, but his experience in biological research played an essential role in his own development as a thinker. Over a quarter of his writings were on biology, and his biological work was crucial in distancing him from his teacher, Plato.[30] Beyond biology, he was a true universal genius, writing with permanent impact on such subjects as logic, metaphysics, art, theater, psychology, economics, and politics. His dominating influence on the physical and biological sciences, however, largely disappeared in the last several centuries. Perhaps Aristotle's most egregious scientific error fell in the domain we now call neuroscience: he systematically denied the controlling role of the brain in sensation and move-ment, giving this function instead to the heart.

Aristotle was born in 384 BCE in Stageira to a medical family. His father, who had been personal physician to Amyntas II, King of Macedonia (father of Philip II), died at a young age, and Aristotle's early education was probably provided by his father's fellow physicians. In those days, as now, a well-educated physician needed some general culture, so at the age of seventeen he was sent off to Plato's Academy in Athens. He stayed there for twenty years and never did begin his medical training.

When Plato died in 347, his nephew took over the Academy, and Aristotle left Athens with some friends for the island of Lesbos and the adjacent mainland where he apparently spent much time studying marine biology. Philip then appointed him private tutor to his son, Alexander, until, at age sixteen, Alexander became regent of Macedonia and had little time for further academic studies. Aristotle returned to Athens in 335 and founded a new school and research center, the lyceum. It received financial support from Alexander who, according to Pliny, also sent it biological specimens as he proceeded to conquer the known world. Thirteen years later and a few months before his death, Aristotle was driven from Athens by the ascent of anti-Alexandrian factions. Aristotle, or so Diogenes Laertius and other ancient authorities tell us, was small, lisping, sarcastic, arrogant, elegant, and happily married.[31]

Now let us turn to Aristotle's views on the brain, which have embarrassed and puzzled historians and scientists since Galen of Pergamum, who "blushed to quote" them.[32] Aristotle believed that the heart, not the brain, was the center of sensation and movement[33]:

> And of course, the brain is not responsible for any of the sensations at all. The correct view [is] that the seat and source of sensation is the region of the heart. (PA656a)

> . . . the motions of pleasure and pain, and generally all sensation plainly have their source in the heart. (PA666a)

19

. . . all sanguineous animals possess a heart, and both movement and the dominant sense perception originate there. (SW456a)

. . . in all sanguineous animals the supreme organ of the sense-faculties lies in the heart. (YO469a)

Table 1.1 summarizes Aristotle's arguments.

Aristotle was well aware of the earlier claims for the dominance of the brain as opposed to the heart, such as those of Alcmaeon, Plato, and Hippocrates, and repeatedly argues against these "fallacious" views (PA656a, b). For example, he claims his predecessors say that there is a scarcity of flesh around the brain so that sensation can get through. But, Aristotle answers, the fleshlessness is in accordance with the cooling function of the brain; furthermore, the back of the head is also fleshless, but it has no sense organs. The earlier theorists observed that the sense organs are placed near the brain, but Aristotle gives a number of alternative reasons for that. For example, the eyes face forward so that we can see along the line we are moving, and ". . . it is reasonable enough that the eyes should always be located near the brain, for the brain is fluid and cold, and the sense organ of sight is identical in its nature with water." The ears are located on the sides of the head to hear sounds from all directions. In any case, some animals hear and smell but do not have these organs in their head. Furthermore, sense organs are in the head because the blood is especially pure in the head region, which makes for more precise sensation.

Galen and many subsequent historians of medicine were somewhat unfair in maintaining that Aristotle simply dismissed the brain as cold and wet. Rather, for Aristotle the brain was second only to the heart in importance and was essential to the functioning of the heart. In fact, the two formed a unit that controlled the body. The heart, which is naturally hot, he determined, must be counterbalanced, in order to attain the mean, the true and the rational position. Thus, the brain, which is naturally cold, "tempers the heat and seething of the heart" (PA652b):

Table 1.1 Aristotle's Arguments for the Heart and Against the Brain as the Center for Sensation and Movement

Heart	Brain
1. Affected by emotion (PA669a)	1. Not affected (PA652b,656a)
2. All animals have a heart or similar organ (GA771a, PA665b)	2. Only vertebrates and cephalopods have one, and yet other animals have sensations (PA652b)
3. Source of blood which is necessary for sensation (PA667b)	3. Bloodless and therefore without sensation (HA494a, 514a, PA765a)
4. Warm, characteristic of higher life (SS439a)	4. Cold (PA652, HA495a5)
5. Connected with all the sense organs and muscles, via the blood vessels (GA744a, HA492a, 469a, GA781a)	5. Not connected with the sense organs or the connection is irrelevant (PA652b, HA503b)
6. Essential for life (YO469a, PA647a)	6. Not so (HA532a, GA741b)
7. Formed first, and last to stop working (GA741b)	7. Formed second (GA674b)
8. Sensitive (SS439a, PA669a)	8. Insensitive: if the brain of a living animal be laid bare, it may be cut without any signs of pain or struggling (PA652b, 656a)
9. In a central location, appropriate for its central role (PA670a)	9. Not so

For if the brain be either too fluid or too solid, it will not perform its office, but in the one case will freeze the blood and in the other will not cool it at all, and thus, cause disease, madness and death. For the cardiac heart and the center of life is most delicate in its sympathies and is immediately sensitive to the slightest change or affection of the blood or the outer surface of the brain. (PA653b)

Aristotle gave the following explanations for the cold nature of the brain: (a) the blood it contains in its vessels is thin, pure, and easily cooled (SS444a); (b) the vessels on and in the brain are very thin and permit evaporation, cooling the brain (SW458a); and (c) when the brain is boiled and the water in it evaporates, hard earth is left, indicating that the brain is made of water and earth, both of which are intrinsically cold (PA653a). So that the brain does not become completely cold, it receives a moderate amount of heat from branches of the aorta and the vena cava that end in the membrane that surrounds the brain (PA652b). When the brain cools the hot vapor reaching it from the heart, phlegm is produced. This idea that the brain produces phlegm is also found in "On the Sacred Disease," as noted above, and is fossilized in our own word "pituitary," coming from the Latin *pituita,* which means phlegm.

Man's brain, according to Aristotle, is the largest and moistest brain for its size (HA494b, PA653a). This is because man's heart is hottest and richest and must be counterbalanced, for man's superior intelligence depends on the fact that his larger brain is capable of keeping the heart cool enough for optimal mental activity (PA648a, 650b–51a). [Woman's brain is smaller than man's (PA653b), a view of Aristotle's that persisted much longer than his view of the mental functions of the heart.] Thus, Aristotle did not merely dismiss the brain as cold and wet. Indeed, it would have been unlike him to dismiss any organ, as he thought none was made without a function to perform. Rather, he believed the brain played an essential, although subordinate, role in a heart-brain system that was responsible for sensation; indeed, man's superior intelligence is credited to his large brain.

Although Aristotle may have not ignored the brain quite as much as is often claimed, it remains puzzling why he made such a startling error and took such a different view from Alcmaeon and the Hippocratic doctors, and above all from his teacher Plato. Aristotle had adduced anatomical, physiological, comparative, embryological, and introspective evidence for his notion of brain function. But an essential approach was absent, namely, the clinical approach, the study of the brain-injured human. The two champions of the hegemony of the brain, Alcmaeon and Hippocrates, were both practicing physicians. The evidence that both gave in support of their opinions was strictly clinical. Since no evidence of systematic experiments on the brain and nervous system appears until Galen in the second century, the accidents of nature were the only sources of information about the function of the brain. It is hard to conceive of

Aristotle, in the course of his strictly zoological observations and dissections, coming across evidence strongly contradicting his theory of the brain and heart.

It seems clear that he never dissected a human, and of the forty-nine animals he did dissect, from elephant to snail, the majority were cold blooded,[34] as were the two, chameleon and turtle, that he obviously vivisected (HA503b, YO486b). These did indeed have cold and wet brains, and the connections of the sense organs with the heart (blood vessels) might have seemed more prominent than those with the brain (nerves). On the other hand, he dissected enough vertebrate brains to describe the two covering membranes (HA494b, 495a), the two symmetrical halves (PA669b), and a "small hollow" in the middle (HA495a), perhaps the lateral ventricles. Finally, it should be noted that Aristotle never localized such psychological faculties as imagination, reasoning or memory in the heart or any place else, but instead viewed them as activities of the whole organism.

Despite (or perhaps because of) his father's profession, Aristotle at no time seemed interested in medicine or medical writing. Indeed, medicine appears to be one of the few things that did not concern this polymath. And, in the fourth century BCE, the study of the effects of damage to the human brain was the most likely way of reaching a "more correct" conception of the brain than Aristotle had. In fact, one of the few places where he approaches a correct view of brain function is in the rare "clinical" passage quoted above (PA653b), in which he suggests that mental disease follows from a malfunctioning of the brain's cooling functions. As discussed in detail below, 600 years later, Galen's observations of human head injuries led him to perform the first recorded experiments on the brain (using piglets), and his observations of spinal injuries to gladiators led directly to his brilliant series of experiments on the effects of spinal cord transection. Even today, it is often primarily clinical data that inspire experiments on animal brains. Aristotle was a pure biologist, not an applied one, and in his day the methodology of academic biology was incapable of defining the brain's actual role.

Alcmaeon and the Hippocratic doctors' theory of the dominance of the brain in mental life soon prevailed. It was transmitted through Plato's *Timaeus* to the Arab world and then to medieval and Renaissance Europe.[35] Yet,

Aristotle's advocacy of the hegemony of the heart persisted alongside. A common resolution was to combine the two views. For example, the great Arab Aristotelian and physician Ibn Sina (Avicenna) did this by placing sensation, cognition, and movement in the brain, which in turn he believed was controlled by the heart.[36] Similarly, according to the thirteenth-century Hebrew encyclopedist Rabbi Gershon ben Schlomoh d'Arles,[37] the brain and heart share functions, so "when one . . . is missing, the other alone continues its activities . . . by virtue of their partnership." As Scheherazade[38] tells it on the 439th night, when the Caliph's savant asks the brilliant girl Tawaddud, "where is the seat of understanding," she answers, "Allah casteth it in the heart whence its illustrious beams ascend to the brain and there become fixed." And Portia's song in the *Merchant of Venice* asks,

> Tell me where is fancie bred,
> Or in the heart or in the head.

Despite his fallacious understanding of brain function, Aristotle actually facilitated the subsequent development of the study of the brain. At the most general level, his stress on the importance of dissection, coupled with his prestige, encouraged others to carry out anatomical studies.[39] More specifically, he played several roles, albeit indirect ones, in the founding of the great Museum at Alexandria, and it was here that systematic human neuroanatomy started.

The Alexandrians and the Beginning of Human Neuroanatomy

Neither the presocratics nor the Hippocratic doctors referred specifically to the convolutions of the cerebral cortex. The first to do so was Praxagoras of Cos[40] (ca. 300) and his student Philotimos. Praxagoras's primary claim to fame was that he was among the first to distinguish arteries and veins clearly and to use the pulse as a major diagnostic technique. He also referred to the "long flexuosities and winding and folding of the convolutions" of the brain. However, the functions of these convolutions were not considered until the beginning of the study of human anatomy in the Museum at Alexandria.

The museum was founded at the end of the fourth century BCE by Ptolemy I, the first Greek ruler of Egypt. It was a vast state-supported institute for research, perhaps like some combination of the National Institutes of Health and the Institute for Advanced Study or All Souls College. Over 100 professors lived communally and had their salaries and expenses paid by the government. The museum contained lecture and study rooms, an astronomical observatory, a zoo, a botanical garden, and dissecting and operating rooms.[41] Its huge library was named a wonder of the ancient world.

In several ways, the museum was a continuation and expansion of Aristotle's Lyceum.[42] First, Ptolemy I had been a young pupil of Aristotle, along with Alexander. Presumably, Aristotle stressed biology in their tutorials since that was his major interest at the time. Second, Demetrius and Strato, who were both students of Theophrastus, Aristotle's long-term collaborator and his successor as head of the Lyceum, were called to Alexandria by Ptolemy to advise him on the organization of the museum. (Ptolemy tried unsuccessfully to hire Theophrastus himself.) Third, the core of the library's collection is thought to have been gathered by Demetrius, at least in part, from Aristotle's own collection. As Strabo, the first-century historian and geographer, later put it, "Aristotle taught the kings of Egypt how to organize a library."[43]

Thus, it was in the shadow of Aristotle that the great museum anatomists, Herophilus (ca. 270) and then Erasistratus (ca. 260), began the systematic study of the structure of the human body.[44] The immediate cause of this extraordinary surge in anatomy in second-century Alexandria was that it was the first time and place in which open dissection of the human body could be carried out. Previously, dissections had been done only on animals. The Greek reverence (and dread) of the dead human body had made its dissection quite impossible. What made Alexandria different? A number of factors seem to have come together.[45]

One was that Herophilus and Erasistratus had the full support of a totalitarian regime determined to glorify itself through the achievement of its scientists. As absolute rulers in a foreign land, the Ptolemys brought few inhibitions with them. A second factor must have been that dissection of the human body for the purposes of mummification had been practiced in Egypt for centuries, and thus the general cultural background undoubtedly helped make human dissection possible. However, it is very unlikely that Greek anatomists had any contact with Egyptian embalmers, as the social gap between the Greeks in Alexandria and the natives surrounding them seems to have been enormous.[46] Another factor may have been changes in philosophical attitudes toward dying and the human corpse that were becoming common by this time: Aristotle had taught that after death the body was no more than a physical frame without feeling or rights.

The uniqueness of the Alexandria-anatomy nexus is revealed by the fact that not only was human dissection first practiced in that city, but this was the first and virtually the only place where human vivisection was systematically carried out for scientific purposes.[47] As Celsus, the Roman historian of medicine, put it[48]:

> It is therefore necessary [for medical students] to dissect the bodies of the dead and examine their viscera and intestines. Herophilus and Erasistratus, they say, did this in the best way by far when they cut open men who were alive, criminals out of prisons, received from kings. And while breath still remained in these criminals, they inspected those parts which nature previously had concealed . . . Nor is it cruel, as most people maintain, that remedies for innocent people of all times should be sought in the sacrifice of people guilty of crimes, and only a few such people at that.

Vivisection of humans for scientific research was never systematically practiced again until the Germans and Japanese did it in World War II. Even the dissection of human cadavers disappeared in the West until it was revived in the new medieval universities in the thirteenth century, and then initially only for forensic, not medical or scientific, purposes.[49]

Both Herophilus and Erasistratus were particularly interested in the brain. They provided the first detailed, accurate descriptions of the human brain including the ventricles.[50] Like Alcmaeon and the Hippocratic doctors before them, they had no question about the brain's dominant role in sensation, thought, and movement.

Herophilus claimed that the fourth ventricle was the "command center," a view later rejected by Galen,[51] who stressed the importance of brain tissue itself. Herophilus compared the cavity in the posterior floor of the fourth ventricle with the cavities in the pens that were in use in Alexandria at the time, and it is still called calamus scriptorius, "reed pen," or sometimes calamus Herophili.

Erasistratus likened the convolutions of the brain to the coils of the small intestine, a comparison that persisted into the nineteenth century, often with Erasistratus's name still attached. Indeed, in the nineteenth century the cerebral convolutions were often called the "enteroid processes," and many drawings of the cortex looked more like the small intestine than like the brain[52] (see figures 1.13 and 1.14). Erasistratus compared the brain convolutions of a number of animals, including hares and stags, with those of humans. From these comparisons, he attributed the greater intelligence of humans to their more numerous convolutions. Galen[53] later ridiculed Erasistratus's correlation between intelligence and the number of convolutions by noting that a donkey had more brain convolutions than humans. However, Galen and possibly Erasistratus may have been referring to the convolutions of the cerebellum rather than those of the cerebrum. In any case, Galen's sarcasm had an extraordinarily pervasive influence and was repeatedly quoted over the next 1500 years, by Vesalius (1543) among others. It seemed to have inhibited any serious interest in the cerebral convolutions until Willis in the seventeenth century.

Erasistratus traced both sensory and motor nerves into the brain and was reported to have made experiments on the living brain to determine its functions, but no accounts of this work survive. He certainly had a understanding of the nature of research, as reflected in this quotation from his work *On Paralysis*[54]:

Those who are completely unused to inquiry are in the first exercise of their mind, blinded and dazed and straightway leave off the inquiry from mental fatigue and an incapacity that is no less than that of those who enter races without being used to them. But the man who is used to inquiry tries every possible loophole as he conducts his research and turns in every direction and so far from giving up the inquiry in the space of a day, does not cease his search throughout his life.

After Herophilos and Erasistratus Alexandrian medicine declined rapidly into various schools that fought over arcane medical theory.[55]

Galen of Pergamon, Prince of Physicians

Galen (129–199 CE) was the most important figure in ancient medical science and is our best source of information about it. He represents its peak; it was through his eyes that the medieval world saw the human body, and that today we see the panorama of classical anatomy, physiology, and medicine.[56] His principal writings (figure 1.5) on the brain that have been translated into English are in *On the Usefulness of the Parts of the Body, On Anatomical Procedures,* and *On the Doctrines of Plato and Hippocrates.*[57]

Galen provided an accurate and detailed account of the anatomy of the brain. Indeed, quite how accurate was not appreciated until recently, when neurohistorians realized that his descriptions fit the brain of the then much more available ox than they do that of the human.[58] He described the ventricles in considerable detail because they were crucial in his physiological system. The ventricles were the site of storage of psychic pneuma (animal spirits), which was the active principle of both sensory and motor nerves and the central nervous system.

On the basis of his extensive clinical experience at the gladiatorial school in Pergamon, Galen distinguished sensory and motor nerves. He believed the former traveled to the anterior part of the brain and the latter came from the posterior part, a clear anticipation of Müller's doctrine of specific nerve energies (the idea that the functions of a nerve are determined by its central connections). He viewed sensation as a central process, since he knew from his clinical data as well from his animal experiments that sensation could be impaired by brain injury even when the sense organs were intact.

Although the ventricles, particularly the anterior ventricle, were important as a source of psychic pneuma, Galen located the soul not there but in the solid portions of the brain. Among the arguments for this was his demonstration that when brain lesions penetrated to the ventricles, death did not invariably result even if both sensation and movement were lost. Thus, he placed both the soul and higher cognitive functions in the solid portions. Regardless, he ridiculed Erasistratus's correlation between intelligence and the number of brain convolutions, with amazingly long-lasting effects, as mentioned above.

Galen described the optic chiasm and tract, and observed that the tract was "intimately and firmly connected . . . with a part of the brain of a peculiar kind, different in boundaries and circumference from the other parts," presumably the lateral geniculate body. He thought that the optic nerves originated in "the anterior part of the lateral ventricles" (figure 1.6) and noted that experimental pressure on this region of the anterior ventricle resulted in blindness.

A number of Galen's experiments concerned the effects on behavior of experimental lesions of both the central and the peripheral nervous system. Perhaps the most famous was his demonstration that section of the recurrent laryngeal nerve eliminates the ability of a pig to vocalize. This experiment is illustrated in the bottom panel of the frontispiece to the sixteenth-century collection of his works shown in figure 1.5.

At about the time of Galen's death in 199, Greek science and medicine died. People preferred to believe than to discuss, critical faculty gave way to dogma, interest in this world declined in favor of the world to come, and worldly remedies were replaced by prayer and exorcism.

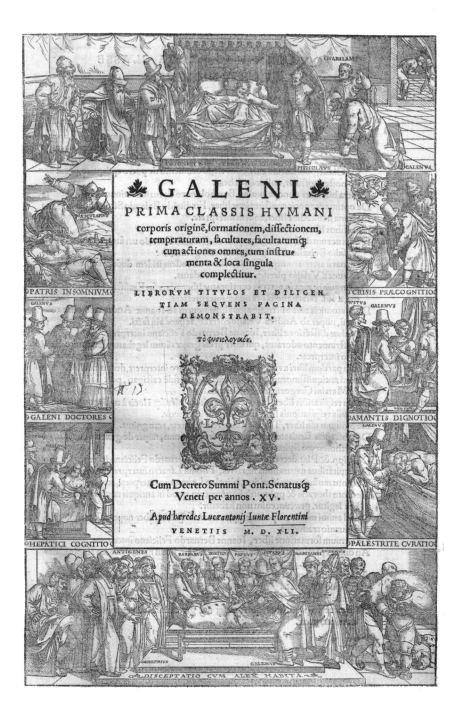

❧ GALENI ❧
PRIMA CLASSIS HVMANI
corporis originē, formationem, diſſectionem,
temperaturam, facultates, facultatumq̃
cum actiones omnes, tum inſtru=
menta & loca ſingula
complectitur.

*LIBRORVM TITVLOS ET DILIGEN
TIAM SEQVENS PAGINA
DEMONSTRABIT.*

τὸ φυσιολογικόν.

Cum Decreto Summi Pont. Senatusq̃
Veneti per annos . XV.
Apud hæredes Lucæantonij Iuntæ Florentini
VENETIIS   M. D. XLI.

THE MEDIEVAL CELL DOCTRINE OF BRAIN FUNCTION

The central feature of the medieval view of the brain was the localization of mental faculties in the organ's ventricles. In its basic form, the faculties of the mind (derived from Aristotle) were distributed among the spaces within the brain (the ventricles described by Galen). The lateral ventricles were collapsed into one space, the first "cell" or small room. It received input from all the sense organs and was the site of the *sensus communis,* or common sense that integrated across the modalities. The sensations yielded images, and thus, fantasy and imagination were often located here too. The second or middle cell was the site of cognitive processes: reasoning, judgment, and thought. The third cell or ventricle was the site of memory (figure 1.7).

Although the basic doctrine remained intact for about 1200 years, there were some minor developments.[59] By the tenth century the original static localization shifted to a more dynamic process analogous to digestion. Sensory inputs were made into images in the first cell and were then transferred to the second cell, whose central location made it warmer, appropriate for further processing (cf. digestion) into cognition. Leftover thoughts were then trans-

Figure 1.5   Title page of the *Omnia Opera* of Galen published in 1541 in Venice. Among the famous anatomists who edited parts of this edition were John Caius, first Master of Gonville and Caius College, Cambridge; John Linacre, founder of the Royal College of Physicians; Jacob Syvius, Vesalius's teacher in Paris and later his archrival; and Vesalius himself, who edited the centrally important *On Anatomical Procedures,* among other Galenic works in the collection.

The eight scenes clockwise from the top are Galen removing his hat and bowing to a distinguished patient; Galen predicting the crisis in a patient's illness; Galen diagnosing lovesickness, which presumably refers to a case in which he revealed sophisticated understanding of the diagnosis of this malady (Mesulam and Perry, 1972); Galen bleeding a patient; Galen's brilliant demonstration in the pig that cutting the recurrent laryngeal nerve eliminates vocalization (among the dignitaries watching is Boethus, an ex-consul who once commissioned an account of this experiment) (Gross, 1998); Galen palpating the liver; Galen and his teachers; and Aesculapius, in a dream, urging Galen's father to send him to medical school. (Courtesy of Yale University, Harvey Cushing/John Hay Whitney Medical Library.)

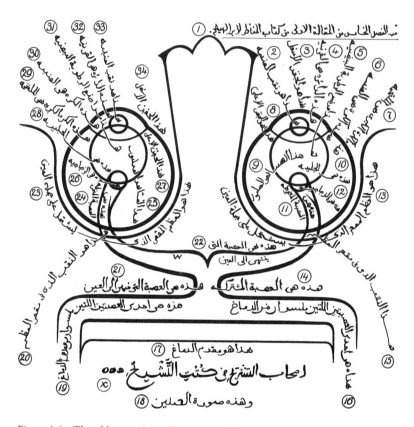

Figure 1.6   The oldest surviving illustration of the eye and visual system, from Ibn al-Haythem's (965–1039) *Book of Optics,* from a copy made in 1083, recopied and labeled by Polyak (1941). Since neither al-Haythem nor earlier Arab medical scientists practiced dissection, and since the content of this diagram is so consistent with Galen's description, Polyak suggests that it is a copy of a Greek original by or derived from Galen. Some of the keys to the numbers: 17, "the anterior portion of the brain"; 16, 19, "one of the two nerves which arise from the anterior portion of the brain"; 14, "the joining [associating] nerve" (i.e., optic chiasm); 21, 22, "the nerve which terminates in the eye." Al-Haythem was known in Europe as Alhazen and the Latin version of his *Book of Optics* (*De Aspectibus*), published in 1572, was the most influential treatise on physiological optics in Europe for at least the next 200 years (Gross, 1981).

ANIMAE· SENSITIVAE

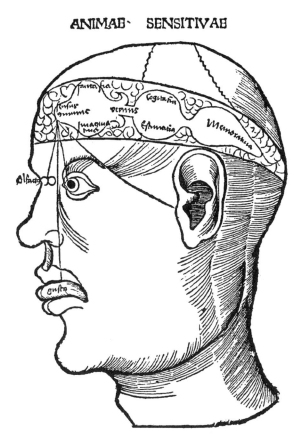

Figure 1.7 The organs of the "sensitive soul" (*anima sensitiva*) from G. Reisch (1503), *Margarita Philosophica* (*Pearls of Philosophy*), one of the first modern encyclopedias. This illustration of ventricular doctrine was copied by many subsequent illustrators as may be seen in the many versions in Clarke and Dewhurst (1996). Messages from the organs of smelling, tasting, seeing, and hearing are united in the common sense (*sensus communis*) in the first ventricle, in which fantasy (*fantasia*) and imagination (*imaginativa*) also reside. The first ventricle communicates with the second by the vermis. Thought (*cogitativa*) and judgment (*estimativa*) are located in the second ventricle. Memory (*memoria*) is in the third ventricle. The curlicues around the ventricles may represent cerebral convolutions. As described in the text, Vesalius ridiculed this particular figure.

ferred to the third cell for storage. These transfers of information occurred through passages between the ventricles that had been described by Galen. Another shift was in the quality of the drawings of the heads in which the ventricles lay, from the crude medieval conceptual representations to the sophisticated pictorial representations of the Renaissance by such masters as Durer and Leonardo (see chapter 2).

How did the cell doctrine arise and why was it so attractive to the medieval and early Renaissance mind? It developed out of a curious amalgam of Greek medical theory and practice and ideological concerns of the early church fathers. Although Galen had described the ventricles in great detail, he localized the mental faculties in the solid portions of the cerebrum. The fourth-century Byzantine Poseidonus developed this idea further.[60] He seems to have been the first to report in detail on the effects of localized brain damage in humans. He said that lesions of the anterior brain substance impaired imagination and lesions of the posterior brain impaired memory, but damage to the middle ventricle produced deficits in reasoning.

The early church fathers were very much concerned with the nonmaterial nature of the soul. Therefore, rather than localize the soul, they localized Aristotle's classification of its functions, namely, those of the mind such as sensation and memory. Furthermore, they believed that brain tissue was too earthy, too dirty to act as an intermediary between the body and soul, so they located mental faculties in the ventricles, empty spaces of the brain. Thus, Nemesius, Bishop of Emesia (ca. 390), put all the faculties of the soul into the ventricles, following the same anteroposterior pattern as his contemporary Poseidonus, but making the site of mental faculties entirely ventricular.[61] Besides the desire for a suitable intermediary between the body and noncorporeal soul, another contribution to the doctrine of three brain cells may have been a parallel with the Trinity.

The three stages of processing postulated for the three cells were also influenced, or at least rationalized, by a comparison with the spatial division of function in classical law courts, as in the following quotation from the *Anatomia*

Nicolai Physici, a twelfth-century text derived from an Islamic synthesis of Nemesius and Poseidonus with Greek humoral and pneumatic physiology[62]:

> On the account of the three divisions of the brain the ancient philosophers called it the temple of the spirit, for the ancients had three chambers in their temples: first the vestibulum, then the consistorium, finally the apotheca. In the first, the declarations were made in law-cases; in the second, the statements were sifted; in the third, final sentence was laid down. The ancients said that the same processes occur in the temple of the spirit, that is, the brain. First, we gather ideas into the cellular phantisca, in the second cell, we think them over, in the third, we lay down our thought, that is, we commit to memory.

The specific placement in the anterior and posterior cells clearly derives from Galen. As noted above, Galen had put sensory processing in the soft and impressionable anterior regions. He thought the posterior portions were motor in function and therefore hard, in order to be able to move muscles. The early church fathers choose this hard region as a good one for the safe storage of valuable brain goods, that is, memories.

Empirical support for the cell doctrine was not lacking, as shown in this quotation from Andre du Laurens (ca. 1597), professor of medicine and chancellor of Montpellier University and physician to Henry IV[63]:

> If we will (saith Aristotle in his Problemes) enter into any serious and deepe conceit we knit the browes and draw them up: if we will call to mind and remember anything, wee hang downe the head, and rub the hinder part, which sheweth very well that the imagination lieth before and the memorie behinde . . . in the diverse pettie chambers in the braine, which the Anatomists call ventricles . . .

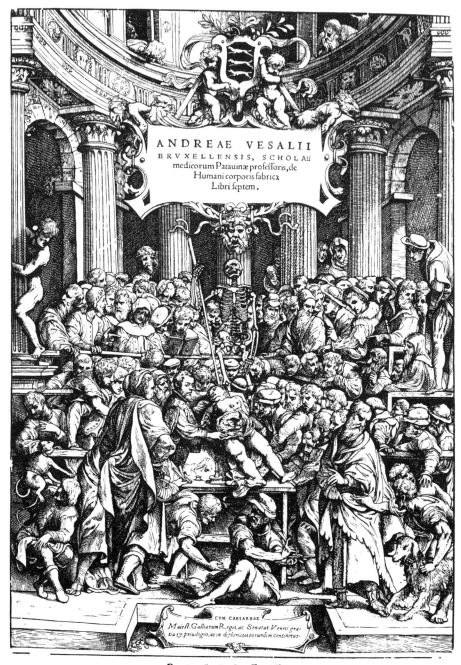

BASILEAE.

THE REBIRTH OF BRAIN SCIENCE

Vesalius Resurrects Neuroanatomy

Andreas Vesalius of Padua (1514–1564) was the greatest of the Renaissance anatomists: he rekindled anatomical science and virtually broke Galen's stranglehold on the field. He is often paired with Copernicus as an initiator of the scientific revolution. In his *De Humani Corporis Fabrica* (1543), the study

Figure 1.8   Title page of Andreas Vesalius's *De Humani Corporis Fabrica* (1543) and one of the most striking and famous woodcuts of the fourteenth century. Until the nineteenth century, the artist was usually thought to be Titian, but modern scholarship suggests that he was a member of Titian's workshop. In any case the engraver of this and the other plates must have been closely supervised by Vesalius. This very busy scene contains many symbols and details of Vesalius's times and work (O'Malley, 1964; Saunders and O'Malley, 1950).

It is a public dissection conducted by Vesalius, recognizable in the center from his portrait. Unlike the custom of the time (see figure 1.9), Vesalius is dissecting with his own hands. His assistant, shown below the table, is relegated to sharpening his knives. Such dissections were required by the statutes of the University of Padua. The bodies, usually male, were obtained from executions, which the courts often spaced out for the convenience of the dissections. This woman tried to escape the hangman by claiming pregnancy, but midwives denied her claim. The dissection is being held outdoors in front of an imaginary Palladian building, with a temporary wooden structure for the spectators that was customary until 1584 when dissections were moved indoors. Ten years later, a permanent dissecting theater was built, which can still be visited in Padua.

Vesalius is surrounded by representatives of the university, the city, the church, and the nobility, as well as by other doctors and students. The toga-clad symbols of classical medicine are shown on the same level as Vesalius. Galen's use of animals is symbolized by the monkey on the left and the dog on the right. The central skeleton represents the importance Vesalius gave skeletal anatomy. Such articulated skeletons, including ones of animals and of humans on horseback, were common fixtures of the anatomical theaters of the time. The bearded figure to the right of the skeleton is wearing Jewish clothing and perhaps is Lazarus de Frieis, a Jewish physician and friend of Vesalius.[64] The nude on the left reflects the importance of surface anatomy for Vesalius. The decorations at the top include the lion of Venice (of which Padua was a part), the ox head of the University of Padua, Vesalius's crest, three sables courant, and the monogram of the publisher, Johannes Oporinus.[65]

of nature, particularly the nature of humanness, begins again in the West and, by implication, dependence on church-sanctified authority for knowledge is rejected. The teaching of anatomy by Vesalius is illustrated in figure 1.8 and before Vesalius in figure 1.9.

Figure 1.10 shows one of Vesalius's famous and beautiful drawings of a horizontal dissection of the human brain. Vesalius ridiculed the ventricular doctrine of brain function, writing with regard to Reisch's representation, "Such are the inventions of those who never look into our maker's ingenuity in the building of the human body."[66] His principal argument against placing the functions of the soul in the ventricles was that many animals have ventricles similar to those in humans and yet they are denied a reigning soul. Indeed, he so equated human and animal brains that he was opposed to vivisection of the brain in animals because "it would be guilty of depriving brute creatures of memory, reason and thought as their structure is the same as that of man."

As to the true functions of the ventricles, he commented[67]:

I believe nothing ought to be said of the locations of the faculties . . . of the principle soul in the brain—even though they are so assigned by those who today rejoice in the name of theologians.

Despite this skepticism about the importance of the ventricles, note that Vesalius drew and labeled the ventricular structures in much more detail and with much more care than he depicted the cerebral cortex.

Ventricular localizations continued among both scientific and lay writers. Perhaps the most recent attribution of important cognitive function to the ventricles by a major scientist was Sir Richard Owen's attempt, in the middle of the nineteenth century, to find the uniqueness of humans in their supposed unique ventricular structures, particularly the hippocampus minor. (See chapter 4.) The most famous lay mention of ventricles is certainly Shakespeare's in *Love's Labours Lost* (IV, ii, 68):

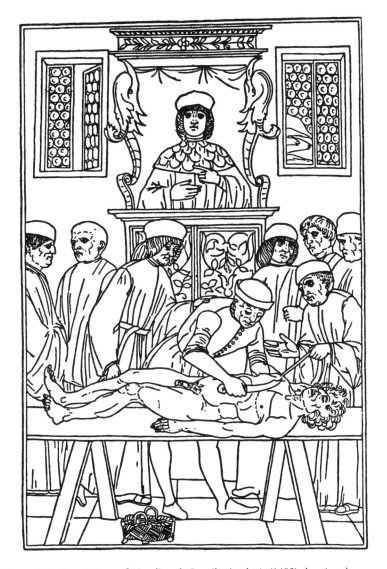

Figure 1.9 Frontispiece of Mondino de Luzzi's *Anothmia* (1493) showing the teaching of anatomy in the fifteenth century. The professor in his academic robes and in his academic chair reads from Galen, or perhaps in this case from Mondino, an *ostensor* or teaching assistant directs with a pointer, and the menial *demonstrator* actually dissects. The students standing around in academic dress are supposed to be observing but not dissecting. This work was the first European anatomy textbook; its first edition was unillustrated, written in 1316. It was essentially a guide for learning Arabic accounts of Galen rather than for actual dissection of the human body.

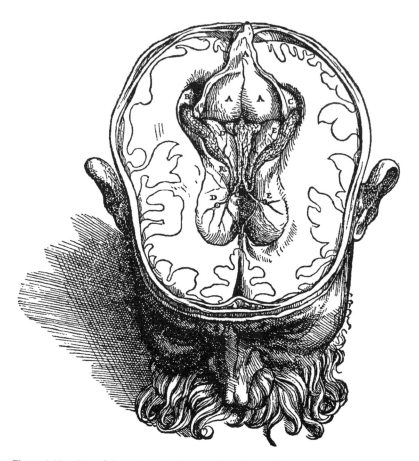

Figure 1.10   One of the series of horizontal dissections of the brain from Vesalius (1543). The fornix (A) has been retracted. Note how the various ventricular structures have been drawn and labeled in detail, but the cortex is drawn in a rudimentary fashion.

A foolish extravagant spirit, full of forms, figures, shapes, objects,
ideas, apprehensions, motions, revolutions. They are begat in the
ventricle of memory, nourished in the womb of pia mater.

Turning to the convolutions, Vesalius pointed out, you "may learn the
shape of these twistings by observing the brain of some animals [on your plate]
at breakfast or at dinner." He agreed that Galen was correct in rejecting
Erasistratus's correlation of their number with intelligence; he believed their
true function was to allow the blood vessels to bring nutriment to the deeper
parts of the brain.[68]

Cerebral Cortex: Gland or Rind?

The first clear distinction between the cerebral cortex and white matter was
made by Archiangelo Piccolomini (1526–1586), professor of anatomy in Rome,
who succeeded in separating the two in gross dissection. He called the former
cerebrum and the latter medulla, and noticed "certain lines" in the cerebrum.[69]
The terms cortex (or rind), substantia cineretia (or brown substance), convolutions, and cerebrum continued to be used interchangeably into the nineteenth
century. Medullary substance also continued to be a synonym for white matter.
As reflected in the word "rind," most workers attributed little importance to
the cortex.

Marcello Malpighi (1628–1694), professor in Bologna, the founder of
microscopic anatomy and discoverer of capillaries, was the first to examine the
cortex microscopically. He saw it as made up of little glands with attached ducts
(figure 1.11). Similar globules were reported by Leeuwenhoek and many
subsequent microscopists.[70] Perhaps they were observing pyramidal cells.[71] At
least in Malpighi's case, artifact is a more likely possibility, since his globules
were more prominent in boiled than fresh tissues.[72] Malpighi's theory of the
brain as a glandular organ was commonly held in the seventeenth and eighteenth centuries, perhaps because it fit with the much earlier, but still persisting,

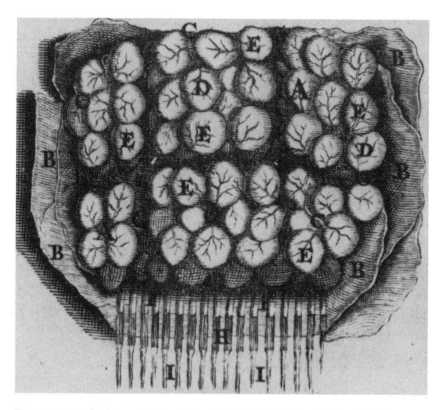

Figure 1.11 Malpighi's cortical glands from his *De Cerebri Cortice* (1666) with their attached fibers. Although he may have seen brain cells, these drawings are likely to be of artifacts as explained in the text. Swedish mystic Swedenborg used these supposed cortical elements to build an elaborate theory of brain function that has close similarities with the neuron doctrine. (See chapter 3.)

Aristotelian concept of the brain as a cooling organ, and the Hippocratic theory that it was the source of phlegm.[73]

The other common view was that the cortex is largely made up of blood vessels. One of the earliest advocates of this was Frederik Ruysch (1628–1731), professor of anatomy in Amsterdam, who noted, "the cortical substance of the cerebrum is not glandular, as many anatomists have described it, nay have positively asserted, but wholly vascular."[74] Here the convolutions were considered mechanisms for protecting the delicate blood vessels of the cortex. Representative of this notion was Thomas Bartholin (1660–1680), professor of anatomy in Copenhagen and discoverer of the lymphatic system. After yet again rejecting Erasistratus's association of the convolutions with intelligence, Bartholin indicated that their true purpose was[75]:

> . . . to make the cerebral vessels safe by guiding them through these tortuosities and so protect them against danger of rupture from violent movements, especially during full moon when the brain swells in the skull.

Thomas Willis Turns Toward Cortex

Before Gall and the development of his phrenological system at the beginning of the nineteenth century, only a very few isolated figures advocated significant functions for the cerebral cortex. The first was Thomas Willis (1621–1675), one of the most important figures in brain science since Galen.[76] Willis was educated at Oxford, quite early gained the Chair of Natural Philosophy there as well as a very lucrative private practice, and was one of the founders of the Royal Society. His *Cerebri Anatomie*[77] was the first monograph on the brain and dealt with physiology, chemistry, and clinical neurology as well as anatomy. Many of its illustrations were by the great architect Sir Christopher Wren, then professor of astronomy at Oxford.

Willis implicated the "cortical and grey part of the cerebrum" in the functions of memory and will. In his scheme, sensory signals came along sensory

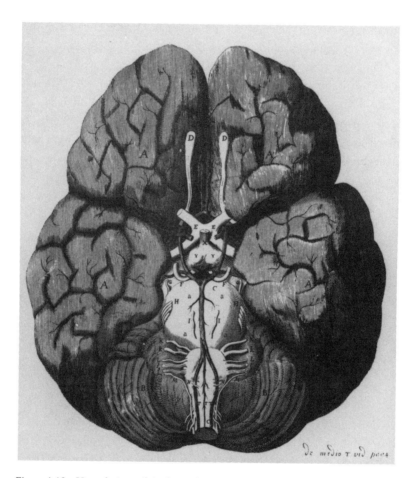

Figure 1.12 Ventral view of the brain from Willis, *Cerebri Anatomie* (1664), drawn
by Christopher Wren. Note the detailed drawing and labeling of the cranial nerves
and basal brain structures (including the circle of Willis) in contrast to the vague
and partially obscured representation of the cerebral cortex, all of which has the single designation A. This schematic and stylized treatment of the cortex was characteristic of all of Willis's illustrations, although he took relatively more interest in
the cortex than most others in the surrounding centuries.

pathways into the corpus striatum, where common sense was located. They were then elaborated into perceptions and imagination in the overlying white matter (then called the corpus callosum or hard body since it was harder than the cortex) and passed to the cerebral cortex where they were stored as memories. In his words[78]:

> As often as a sensible impression, such as a visual stimulus, arrives from the periphery it turns inwards like an undulation of water and is transferred to the corpora striata where the sensation received from outside becomes a perception of internal sense. If, however, this impression is carried further and penetrates the corpus callosum, imagination takes the place of sensation. If after this the same undulation of the spirits strikes against the cortex, as it were the outermost banks, it imprints there a picture or character of the object which, when it is later reflected from there revives the memory of the same thing.

The cortex initiates voluntary movement whereas the cerebellum is involved only in involuntary movement.

Willis's ideas on brain function came not only from his dissections but also from his experiments on animals and correlation of symptoms and pathology in humans. Willis noticed that whereas the cerebellum was similar in a variety of different mammals, the complexity of the cerebral convolutions varied greatly among animals; this variation was correlated with intellectual capacity:

> Hence, these folds or convolutions are far more numerous and rarer in man than in any other animal because of the variety and number of acts of the higher Faculties, but they are varied by a disordered and almost haphazard arrangement so that the operations of the animal function might be free, changeable and not limited to one. Those gyri are fewer in quadrupeds, and in such as the cat, they

are found to have a particular shape and arrangement so that this beast considers or recalls scarcely anything except what the instincts and demands of nature suggest. In the smaller quadrupeds, and also in birds and fish, the surface of the brain is flat . . . Hence it is that animals of this sort understand or learn few things.

Despite the importance of the cerebral cortex in Willis's schema, his work contains no adequate drawing of the cortex; he apparently never asked Wren or anybody else to produce one (figure 1.12). In fact, for another 150 years the cortex continued to be drawn as Erasistratus first suggested: as coils of the small intestine (figures 1.13 and 1.14).

Although Willis was a major figure of his time and beyond, his ideas on the importance of the cerebral cortex fell out of favor, and theories of the cortex as a glandular, vascular, or protective rind returned to their original dominance. Two men, however, did challenge the earlier beliefs. The first was Francois Pourfour du Petit (1644–1741), a French army surgeon.[79] He carried out a series of systematic experiments on the effects of cortical lesions in dogs and related them to his clinicopathological observations in wounded soldiers. From these studies he realized that the cerebral cortex plays a critical role in normal movement and that this influence is a contralateral one. However, his observations were totally ignored until they were rediscovered much later. Perhaps this was because du Petit did not hold an academic post and he published his account in a very limited edition. Yet, his conclusion that the cortex was insensitive to touch was repeatedly cited to support the theories of von Haller who, as discussed below, was the dominant physiologist of the day. Thus, du Petit's work demonstrating motor functions of cortex was probably ignored largely because of the anticortex ideology of the time, not because it was published in a minor journal.

The second major figure advocating the importance of the cortex between Willis and Gall was Emanuel Swedenborg (1688–1772), founder and mystical prophet of the New Jerusalem or Swedenborgian Church, which is still active in United States and Great Britain. On the basis of reviewing the

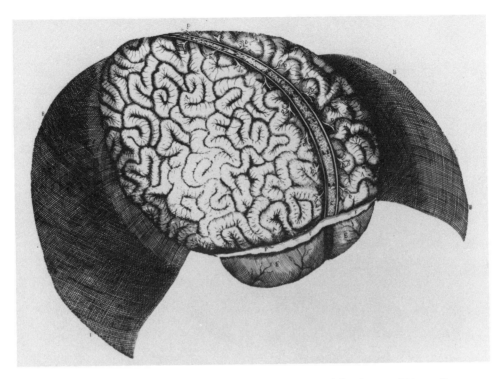

Figure 1.13   The depiction of the cerebral convolutions by Raymond de Viessens of Montpellier, a leading neuroanatomist of the late seventeenth century, in *Neurographia Universalis* (1685). The convolutions are not differentiated in any way and, following Erasistratus, look like intestines.

contemporary literature, Swedenborg arrived at an amazing set of prescient ideas on the importance of the cerebral cortex in sensation, cognition, and movement. The nature of these ideas and why they remained essentially unknown until the twentieth century are discussed in chapter 3.

Von Haller and the Insensitivity of Cortex

The space we have given to Willis, du Petit, and Swedenborg, men who thought the cortex was a crucial brain structure, is somewhat misleading since

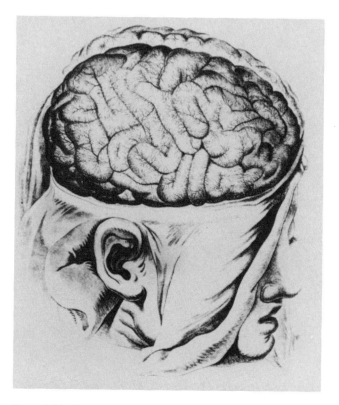

Figure 1.14 In Vicq d'Azyr's *Traite d'Anatomie et Physiologie* (1786)
the convolutions still are drawn looking like intestines, but now
bear some relation to the actual morphology of the brian.

the opposite view prevailed heavily throughout the 2000 years between Erasistratus and Gall (figure 1.15). Much more representative and influential was
Albrecht von Haller (1708–1777), professor at Tubingen and later Bern, who
dominated physiology in the middle of the eighteenth century.[80] In his monumental *Elementa Physiologiae Corporis Humani* (1757–1765, in eight volumes)
and his *Icones Anatomicae* (1743–1756) he divided the organs of the body, as
well as parts of the nervous system, into those "irritable" (e.g., muscle) and
those "sensible" (e.g., sense organs and nerves). He tested sensibility with

mechanical and chemical stimuli and found the cortex to be completely insensitive. In contrast, he reported that stimulation of the white matter and subcortical structures in experimental animals produced expressions of pain, attempts to escape, or convulsions, thereby demonstrating the sensibility of these structures.

From observations such as these Haller concluded that all parts of the cortex were equivalent because stimulation had the same negative effect, and that all subcortical regions were also equivalent because their stimulation had similar positive effects. Thanks to his prestige and many students and followers, Haller's concept of the insensitivity and equipotentiality of cortex superceded the observations of Willis, Swedenborg, and du Petit, and persisted well into the next century.[81, 82] As to the cortex itself, Haller was of the cortex-as-bloodvessels school[83]:

> . . . the greater part of it consists of mere vessels . . . as to glandules making the fabric . . . that notion has been discarded; nor has there been any opinion received with less probability than this.

Gennari and His Stripe

A few years after Swedenborg died, an event occurred that was particularly central to the theme of this discussion: the discovery of the stripe of Gennari, which we now know marks, in primates, the location of striate cortex—the primary visual cortex. Francisco Gennari (1752–1797), then a medical student, in the course of examining frozen sections of an unstained human brain, observed and reported on a white line in the cortex that was especially prominent and sometimes double in the posterior part of the brain[84] (figure 1.16). This was the first evidence that the cerebral cortex was not uniform in structure. The more famous Vicq d'Azyr[85] rediscovered the stripe and for a while it was known as the stripe of Vicq d'Azyr, until priority was sorted out and the name reverted to Gennari.[86] As to its function, Gennari commented, "Just as the use of so many other things is as yet concealed from us, so I do not know the purpose for which this substance was created."[87]

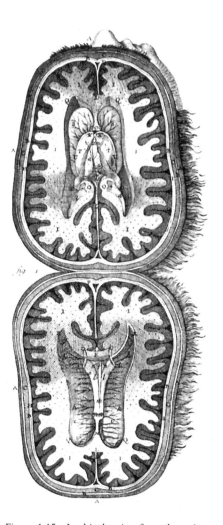

Figure 1.15 In this drawing from the article on anatomy in Diderot's *Encyclopedia,*
note how the ventricular structures are
drawn and labeled in detail, whereas the cortical convolutions are represented schemati-
cally and hardly labeled, reminiscent of
Vesalius's drawing (figure 1.10) 200 years
earlier (Diderot and D'Alembert, 1751).

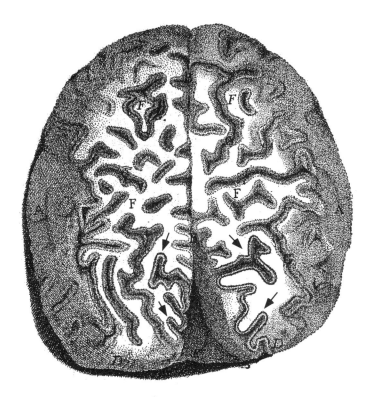

Figure 1.16   In *De Peculiari Structura Cerebri Nonnullisque Eius Morbis* (1782), Gennari was the first to describe regional variations in the structure of the cerebral cortex. Specifically, he noticed a white line in the cortex that is more prominent in the medial and posterior portions of a frozen human brain (arrows added by me). It is now known as the stripe of Gennari.

Gennari never published again, and died a young, penniless compulsive gambler.[88]

THE BEGINNING OF THE MODERN ERA OF CORTICAL LOCALIZATION

Gall and Phrenology

The localization of different psychological functions in different regions of the cerebral cortex begins with Franz Joseph Gall (1758–1828) and his collaborator J. C. Spurzheim (1776–1832), the founders of phrenology.[89] Before they developed their phrenological system, the two men made a number of major neuroanatomical discoveries that would have fixed them in the history of neuroscience even if they had never begun their project of correlating the morphology of the cranium with psychological faculties (figure 1.17). Among Gall's significant anatomical contributions were the recognition that the grey matter is functioning neural tissue connected to the underlying white matter (to which he attributed a conductive function), the first description of postembryonic myelinization, proof of the decussation of the pyramids, the first clear description of the commissures, demonstration that the cranial nerves originate below the cerebrum, and the realization that the brain is folded to conserve space.[90]

The central ideas of their phrenological system were that the brain was an elaborately wired machine for producing behavior, thought, and emotion, and that the cerebral cortex was a set of organs with different functions.[91] They postulated about "thirty-five affective and intellectual faculties" and assumed that (a) these were localized in specific organs of the cerebral cortex; (b) the development or prominence of these faculties was a function of their activity, and the amount of activity would be reflected in the size of the cortical organ; and (c) the size of each cortical organ was indicated by the prominence of the overlying skull, that is, in cranial bumps.

The primary method of data collection used by Gall and Spurzheim was examining the skulls of a great variety of people from lunatics and criminals to

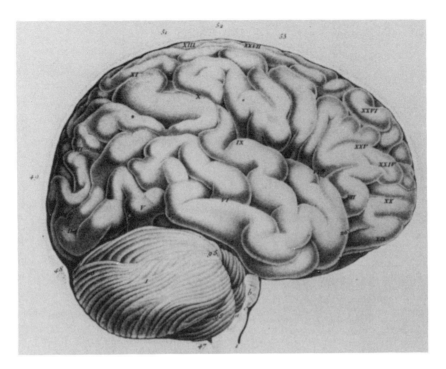

Figure 1.17   This drawing of the cortical convolutions in Gall and Spurzheim's *Anatomie et Physiologie du Systeme Nerveux* (1810) is quite accurate, one of the first to be so. The numbers refer to different phrenological organs.

the eminent and accomplished (figure 1.18). Neuropsychological and animal experimental data, even those gathered by themselves, they considered only minor and ancillary evidence.[92]

Phrenology had wide popular appeal, particularly in England and the United States, and among many leading intellectuals, such as Honoré de Balzac, A. R. Wallace, Horace Mann, and George Eliot.[93] However, it met considerable opposition from the religious, political, and scientific establishments of the day. For example, Gall's public lectures were banned in Austria because they led to materialism and opposed religion and morality. His works were

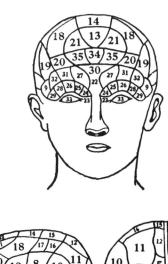

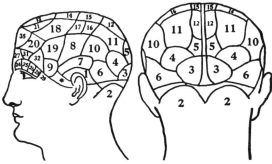

AFFECTIVE FACULTIES		INTELLECTUAL FACULTIES	
PROPENSITIES	SENTIMENTS	PERCEPTIVE	REFLECTIVE
? Desire to live	10 Cautiousness	22 Individuality	34 Comparison
* Alimentiveness	11 Approbativeness	23 Configuration	35 Causality
1 Destructiveness	12 Self-Esteem	24 Size	
2 Amativeness	13 Benevolence	25 Weight and	
3 Philoprogenitiveness	14 Reverence	Resistance	
4 Adhesiveness	15 Firmness	26 Coloring	
5 Inhabitiveness	16 Conscientiousness	27 Locality	
6 Combativeness	17 Hope	28 Order	
7 Secretiveness	18 Marvelousness	29 Calculation	
8 Acquisitiveness	19 Ideality	30 Eventuality	
9 Constructiveness	20 Mirthfulness	31 Time	
	21 Imitation	32 Tune	
		33 Language	

---

placed on the Index of the Catholic Church for similar reasons. In 1908 the French Institute, later the Academy of Science, under the leadership of the great Cuvier, totally rejected even the anatomical parts of a paper that Gall submitted.

Flourens Attacks Gall, but the Cortex (Re)emerges as a Higher Structure

In the scientific world the most important and influential critique of Gall came from Pierre Flourens (1794–1867), later professor of natural history at the Sorbonne.[94] A technically brilliant experimenter, Flourens quickly rose in the French scientific establishment and at the age of thirty-five was elected to the Academy that had rejected Gall. Starting in the 1820s and continuing for over twenty years, he carried out a series of experiments on the behavioral effects of brain lesions, particularly with pigeons. Flourens reported that lesions of the cerebral hemispheres had devastating effects on willing, judging, remembering, and perceiving. However, the site of a lesion was irrelevant: all regions of the hemispheres contributed to these functions. The only exception was vision, in that a unilateral lesion produced only contralateral blindness, but again there was no localization within the hemisphere. These holistic results tended to eclipse Gall's ideas of punctate localization, but only in scientific circles and only temporarily.

Flourens's finding of cognitive losses after hemispheric lesions was actually a confirmation of Gall's emphasis on the cognitive role of the cortex, a concept that had been virtually absent before Gall. This change in attitude toward the cortex was reflected in mid-nineteenth-century textbooks that now routinely attributed intellectual function to the cortex. William Carpenter, in his authoritative *Principles of Human Physiology,*[95] wrote that the convolutions of the cerebrum were:

Figure 1.18 Frontispiece and its legend from J. G. Spurzheim's *Phrenology or the Doctrine of the Mental Phenomenon* (1834). Note that none of the faculties were sensory or motor, but were all "higher" ones.

... the centre of intellectual action ... the site of ideas ... restricted to intellectual operations ... the sole instrument of intelligence ... It is probably by them alone that ideas ... of surrounding objects are acquired ... and that these ideas are made the groundwork of mental operations ... that would also seem to be the exclusive seat of Memory ... and Will.

The cortex was termed a "superadded" structure lying hierarchically and physically above the highest sensory structure, the thalamus, and the highest motor structure, the corpus striatum (figure 1.19). The general idea that the thalamus had major sensory functions and the corpus striatum major motor functions was generally accepted by the middle of the nineteenth century on the basis of a number of studies that traced sensory and motor tracts from the periphery and made experimental lesions in animals.[96]

This view of the higher functions of the cortex, common for the period, combined Haller's notion of insensitivity and both Gall's and Flouren's attribution of higher faculties, but neither sensory nor motor functions, to the cortex.

Broca Confirms Gall

Despite the bitter attacks by Flourens, Gall's theory of punctate localization, and even many of his specific localizations such as language in the frontal lobes and sexuality in the cerebellum, continued to be actively debated in the middle of the nineteenth century.[97] At least in the scientific community, the supposed correlations between skull and brain morphology were quickly recognized as erroneous. Yet, Gall's ideas stimulated the search for correlations between the site of brain injury and specific psychological deficits in patients as well as in experimental animals. Reports of such correlations were published in both the phrenological and mainstream neurological literature, and the question of the localization of psychological function in the brain was hotly debated at scientific meetings.

Thus, in 1848, J. B. Bouillard (1796–1881), professor at la Charité in Paris and a powerful figure in the medical establishment,[98] offered a cash prize for a patient with major frontal lobe damage who did *not* have a language deficit. The debate about localization reached a climax at a series of meetings of the Paris Société d'Anthropologie in 1861. At the April meeting, Paul Broca (1824–1880), professor of pathology at the Sorbonne and founder of the society, announced that he had a critical case on this issue. A patient with long-standing language difficulties—nicknamed "Tan" because that was all that he could say—had just died. The next day Broca displayed his brain at the meeting, and indeed it had widespread damage in the left frontal lobe. Over the next few months he presented several similar cases. Not only did these cases finally establish the principle of discrete localization of psychological function in the brain, but the discovery was hailed as a vindication of Gall. Broca himself regarded Gall's work as "the starting point for every discovery in cerebral physiology in our century."[99]

Evolution and Brain Function

Contributing to the growing interest in the cerebral cortex were ideas about organic evolution that were in the air in the decades before the publication of Darwin's *Origin of Species* (1861). In J.B. Lamarck's (1809) theory of evolution, the first coherent one, evolution involved continuous upward progress, the inevitable transformation of lower into upper forms. The anonymous and widely influential best-seller *Vestiges of the Natural History of Creation* (1844) took a similar progressive view of evolution. (See chapter 4.)

Herbert Spencer (1820–1903) was the first and most important figure to apply evolutionary ideas to the nervous system and psychology.[100] Spencer had virtually no formal education, but read widely in the sciences as a boy. A seminal experience at age 11 was hearing a lecture on phrenology by Spurzheim, and it was decades before he decisively parted from a phrenological position. Before he did so he published in phrenological journals and invented a more accurate device for measuring skull bumps. After a few years as a railway

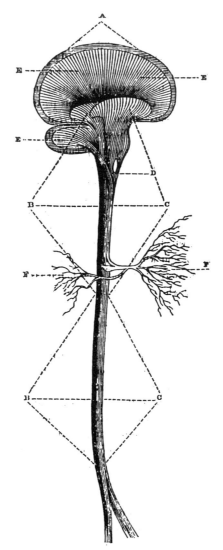

A. The cortical substance or mental portion.
B. B. The sensitive column.   C. C. The motor column.
D. The passage of motor fibres to the cerebellum.
E. E. E. Fibres of volition and consciousness.
F. F. Sensitive and motor fibres.

engineer he drifted into political journalism, where he came into contact with T. H. Huxley, Thomas Carlyle, and George Henry Lewis (and, to use a modern but particularly apt expression, Lewis's partner, George Eliot), and was exposed to the scientific and political issues of the day.

In his first book, *Social Statics* (1851), Spencer set out a quasi-Lamarckian progressive theory of evolution. He argued that it justified survival of the fittest (a phrase Darwin later adopted) in human society. This led him to oppose such things as government help for the poor, public health, and public education. These views were the theoretical bases of the ultraindividualist and conservative ideology that later became known as social Darwinism, although Spencerism would have been a more appropriate designation.[101] Spencer's social theories were particularly welcome among the elites in postbellum America. As John D. Rockefeller put it in a Sunday school address[102]:

> The growth of a large business is merely survival of the fittest. . . . The American beauty rose can be produced in the splendor and fragrance which bring cheer to its beholder only by sacrificing the early buds which grow up around it. This is not an evil tendency in business. It is merely the working-out of a law of nature and a law of God.

In his next work, *Principles of Psychology* (1855), Spencer combined association psychology with evolutionary theory to produce "evolutionary associationism." From evolution he took the idea of a progressive increase in the complexity of the nervous system both phylogenetically and ontogenetically. This led to the conception of the cortex as the newest, highest, and most important level of the nervous system. Furthermore Spencer posited that

Figure 1.19 This figure from a 1837 dissertation illustrates the prevailing view at this time that the highest sensory and motor structures were subcortical (the thalamus and the striatum, respectively, although not so labeled here), and only the cortex had mental functions (Bennett, 1837).

function must be localized in the cortex just as it clearly is in lower nervous structures[103]:

> But no physiologist who calmly considers the question . . . can long resist the conviction that different parts of the cerebrum subserve different kinds of mental action. Localization of function is the law of all organization whatever: separateness of duty is universally accompanied with separateness of structure: and it would be marvellous were an exception to exist in the cerebral hemispheres. Let it be granted that the cerebral hemispheres are the seat of higher psychical activities; let it be granted that among these higher psychical activities there are distinctions of kind . . . more or less distinct kinds of psychical activity must be carried out in more or less distinct parts of the cerebral hemispheres. . . . It is proved experimentally, that every bundle of nerve fibers and every ganglion, has a special duty; and that each part of every bundle of nerve fibers and every such ganglion, has a duty still more special. Can it be, then, that in the great hemispherical ganglia alone, this specialization of duty does not hold?

When the *Origin of Species* was published in 1859, Spencer became a enthusiastic follower of Darwin. He set out to unify all knowledge along the principles of Darwinian evolution and attempted to do so in his massive, multivolume *Principles of Synthetic Philosophy*. Today, his synthetic philosophy is all but forgotten, whereas the disastrous consequences of his social views are still reverberating. However, Spencer did make one permanent and major contribution to modern neuroscience. That was the profound influence of his views of the evolution of the nervous system on John Hughlings Jackson.

John Hughlings Jackson (1835–1911) is the perennial holder of the title, "father of English neurology." As a medical student in Yorkshire, he was so enthralled with Spencer's writings that he almost abandoned medicine to pursue their study full time. Instead, he spent forty-five years as a clinical neurologist at the National Hospital, Queen Square, London, applying Spencer's ideas on the evolution and dissolution of the nervous system. Many of his over 300 papers began with such sentiments as "I should say that a very great part of this paper is nothing more than the application of certain of Herbert Spencer's principles."

Spencer taught that evolution implied a continuity of nervous organization from spinal cord to cerebral cortex. Therefore, as Jackson put it, "If the doctrine of evolution be true, all nervous centers [including the cortex] must be of sensory-motor constitution," that is, they must have both sensory and motor functions.[104] It was the combination of Spencer's theory of cortex as a sensorimotor structure and his insistence on cerebral localization of function, and Jackson's many observations of seizures (including his wife's) that led him to the brilliant clinical inference that the seizures we now call Jacksonian reflect a somototopically organized cortical motor mechanism.

Jackson's ideas on the motor mechanisms of the cerebral cortex were dramatically confirmed in 1870 by Fritsch and Hitsig's demonstration of specific movements from electrical stimulation of the cortex of the dog.[105] These authors were not reticent about the more general implications of their results, as shown by the final lines of their paper:

> It further appears, from the sum of all our experiments . . . certainly some psychological functions and perhaps all of them . . . need certain circumscribed centers of the cortex.

In summary, despite their temporary eclipse under the shadow of Flourens' experiments, Gall's general ideas of punctate localization in the cortex were essentially vindicated by the third quarter of the nineteenth century. By that time, they were considered confirmed by Broca's demonstration of an association between damage to the frontal lobe and aphasia, and again by Fritsch and Hitzig's experiments on stimulation of motor cortex. Gall's ideas on the localization of mental function had a deep and lasting influence through stressing (a) that the human mind could be subdivided into specific functions,

(b) that these specific functions were mediated by discrete brain structures, and (c) that the cerebral cortex was crucially important in mental activity. It is interesting to note that one of the first accurate drawings of the cerebral cortex was by Gall and Spurzheim (figure 1.17). Before them the cortex was often portrayed as a pile of intestines (figures 1.13 and 1.14) or in a crude schematic way with no attention to detail (figure 1.15). Perhaps it is necessary to believe a structure has important functions before one goes to the trouble to portray it accurately.

The Search for Sensory Areas in the Cerebral Cortex

The last quarter of the nineteenth century saw an intense search for the localization of sensory centers in the cortex. In addition to increasing interest in the cortex from the work of Gall, Flourens, Spencer, Jackson, and Fritsch and Hitzig, a major spur to the search for sensory centers was Johannes Müller's doctrine of specific nerve energies.[106] Müller (1801–1858), professor of anatomy and physiology at Berlin, dominated midnineteenth-century physiology through his personality, his many influential students, and his massive *Handbuch der Physiologie* (1833–1840).

Müller's doctrine had three essential elements. The first and most fundamental asserted that sensation was the awareness of the states of sensory nerves, not of the outer world itself. This was a radical departure from the widespread view, derived from the presocratic philosophers Leucippus and Democritus, that images (*eidola*) from objects in the world enter the eye and travel to the brain.[107] The second element was that when a given nerve type or nerve energy was excited, the same type of experience is produced no matter what the stimulus. Thus, photic, mechanical, and electrical stimulation of the eye all produce visual sensations. Müller, following Aristotle, assumed that there were five nerve types or nerve energies; today, we would call them qualities or modalities. The third element of the doctrine was that the same physical stimulus applied to different sense organs gives rise to different sensations. Thus, a blow to the eye and one to the ear produce visual and auditory sensations, respectively.

Müller was unsure of the locus of nerve specificity. As he put it:

It is not known whether the essential cause of the peculiar "energy"
of each nerve of sense is seated in the nerve itself or in the parts
of the brain and spinal cord with which it is connected.

A student of Müller, however, the great Hermann von Helmholtz,
philosopher, physicist, and psychologist, located the specificity squarely in the
nerve terminations. Helmholtz, who was the first to measure the speed of nerve
conduction, in the original comparison of the nervous system with a telegraph
system, noted that with wires[108]:

according to the different kinds of apparatus with which we provide terminations, we can send telegraph despatches, ring bells,
explode mines, decompose water, move magnets, magnetize iron,
develop light and so on. So with the nerves the condition of
excitement which can be produced in them and is conducted in
them, is, so far as can be recognized in isolated fibres of a nerve,
everywhere the same, but when it is brought to various parts of
the brain, or the body, it produces motion, secretions of glands,
increase and decrease of the quantity of blood, of redness and of
warmth of individual organs, and also sensations of light, of hearing,
and so forth.

Emil Du Bois-Reymond, another one of Müller's students,[109] his successor in the Berlin Chair, and discoverer of the action potential, went further and
claimed that if it were possible to cross-connect the auditory and optic nerves,
we would see with our ears and hear with our eyes.[110]

The idea that the specificity of nerves derived from their central connections was not new. On the basis of his clinical practice among gladiators in
Pergamon, Galen distinguished between sensory and motor nerves, and proposed that sensory nerves were connected to the anterior part of the brain and
motor nerves to the posterior. Charles Bell (1774–1842), codiscoverer of the

law of spinal roots, or rather, the sensory half of it,[111] extended the idea of specificity inherent in that law to the five senses to yield in 1811 an account of nerve specificity essentially identical to Müller's later published one. As Bell put it[112]:

> the nerves of sense depend for their attributes on the organs of the brain to which they are severally attached . . . the properties of the nerves are derived from their connections with the parts of the brain.

It is important to note that for both Bell and Müller it was not the terminations in the cerebral cortex that conveyed specificity on the sensory nerves. Rather, for both of them, and, as noted above, more generally for almost all the physiologists and anatomists of the first half of the nineteenth century, the cortex still had no sensory (or motor) functions. The main support for this view was still Haller's that since the cortex was insensitive to touch, it could hardly be sensory. Instead, it was believed to be the site of the highest intellectual functions. This notion was often supported both by the phylogenetic correlation of cortical complexity with intelligence and reports of intellectual deficits after cortical lesions. It was clearly also heavily influenced by Gall's ideas. Note that of all the thirty-five faculties that Gall put into the cerebral cortex, none was sensory or motor. Some of Gall's faculties do have sensory sounding names, but on examination they are actually cognitive. For example as to the faculty of color, Gall notes, "I do not mean the simple faculty of seeing or perceiving colors . . . [but rather] distinguishing the relations of colors: the talent for painting."[113]

What turned Müller's doctrine and everybody else's attention toward the possible sensory functions of the cerebral cortex was Fritsch and Hitzig's discovery of motor cortex by electrical stimulation in 1870. This unambiguously demonstrated that the cerebral cortex had more than just higher functions.

Müller's doctrine of specific nerve energies now became directed toward cortex as the locus of specific energies. Thus, under its influence, in the later part of the nineteenth century, (a) neural pathways were traced from the sense organs into the brain to find the specific regions in which they ended; (b) the cortex was divided up into separate centers or organs on the basis of the pattern of its structure, thereby yielding the techniques of cytoarchitectonics and myeloarchitectonics; (c) cortical lesions were made in animals to find the sensory centers, and (d) in close parallel, attempts were made to correlate sensory losses in humans with the site of cortical damage.

The Discovery of a Visual Center in the Cerebral Cortex

Bartolomeo Panizza: The First Claim

The first person to suggest a discrete localization of visual function in the cortex on the basis of systematic investigations was Bartolomeo Panizza (1785–1867), professor of anatomy at Pavia and a follower of Gall.[114] After examining the brains of several patients who became blind after strokes, he attributed vision to the posterior cortex. He then tested this idea by making lesions and enucleations in a number of species and concluded that the occipital region was the crucial one for vision. He also studied the anatomical and behavioral effects of monocular enucleation as a function of age, and concluded that the effects on the brain were more profound in adults than in infants. Panizza's work seems to have been totally ignored at the time. One reason for this may have been because he only published in local journals, those of the Royal Institute of Lombardy of Science, Arts, and Letters; however, these journals were exchanged with those of the Royal Society and presumably other scientific societies.

A more likely reason for the lack of impact of Panizza's work was the prevailing theoretical view of the relative role of cortex and subcortex. As we have indicated, at that time it was thought that the thalamus was the highest sensory center and the basal ganglia the highest motor center. In contrast, the cortex was believed to be concerned not with sensation or movement but with intellectual operations.[115] This view went back at least to Gall, who among his

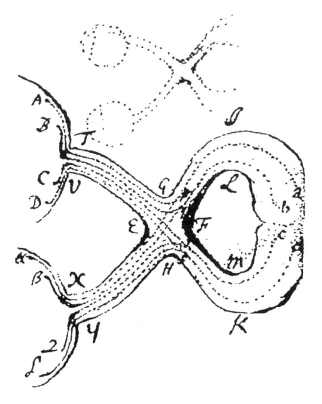

Figure 1.20 Newton (1704) was the first to suggest, in *Opticks,* that partial decussation at the optic chiasm results in binocular convergence. This is clearly and elegantly illustrated in this sketch that Grusser found in Newton's manuscript pages of the *Opticks* (Grusser and Landis, 1991). Note that Newton thought that binocular fusion occurred in the chiasm itself. There is no reason to believe that Newton had any actual anatomical evidence for his model.

thirty-five plus cerebral organs had none for any sensory or motor function. The importance of Panizza's work was realized only after the work of Ferrier, Munk, and Schafer provided convincing evidence for a cortical visual area, as described in the next section.[116]

The Battle for Visual Cortex: Ferrier versus Munk and Schäfer

Immediately after Fritsch and Hitzig's publication, the English physiologist David Ferrier (1843–1928), working at the West Riding Lunatic Asylum and at Kings College, London, confirmed their work, first in dogs and then in monkeys.[117] He then applied their electrical stimulation methods to search for the sensory cortices. He found that stimulation of the angular gyrus (area 7 in posterior parietal cortex) in the monkey produced conjugate eye movements, and he interpreted this as indicating that this area was the seat of the perception of visual impressions. In contrast, he found that stimulation of the occipital lobe or other regions did not have these effects. He further tested this theory by making angular gyrus lesions (figure 1.21) and reported that unilateral lesions produced temporary blindness in the contralateral eye and bilateral lesions produced permanent blindness in both eyes.[118] However, the animals were observed for only a few days before he sacrificed them, the operations having been done without antiseptic techniques. Summarizing the results on four animals with angular gyrus lesions, he wrote:

> The loss of visual perception is the only result of this lesion, the other senses and the powers of voluntary movement being retained so long as the lesion remains confined to the angular gyrus itself. By the term visual perception I wish to indicate the consciousness of visual impressions, and to distinguish this from mere impressions on the optical apparatus and reactions which are only of a reflex nature . . .

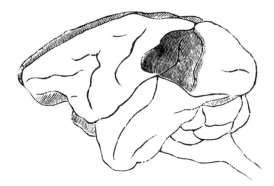

Figure 1.21 Lesions of the angular gyrus in monkeys that Ferrier first claimed produced blindness (1876) and later, only temporary blindness (1886). The lesion comes within a few millimeters of the later-discovered location of the foveal representation in striate cortex. (See figure 1.22.)

In contrast, monkeys with large occipital lesions (figure 1.22) showed no visual disturbances at all unless their lesions encroached on the angular gyrus. The only effect of occipital lesions was a temporary loss of appetite. From this he speculated that the occipital lobes were related to the "organic sensibilities and are the anatomical substrata of the correlated feelings which form a large part of our personality and subjectivity."[119]

How did Ferrier account for the finding that the visual disturbances were evident only through the contralateral eye? Isaac Newton[120] had described the partial decussation of the optic pathways and its significance for binocular vision clearly in his *Opticks* (see figure 1.20) and several other eighteenth-century figures held similar views. Indeed, homonymous hemianopia after unilateral brain damage was explained in terms of partial decussation as early as 1723.[121] Ferrier was aware of both the partial decussation and its possible relation to "hemiopia," as he called it. However, he thought that the uncrossed fibers crossed to the opposite hemisphere at some level beyond the chiasm, so that the cortex of each hemisphere received input from the entire contralateral eye.

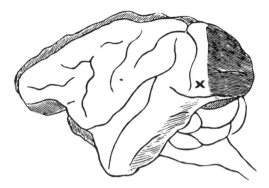

Figure 1.22   Ferrier (1886) found that these occipital
lesions in monkeys do not cause any visual deficits.
The lesion spares part of what we now know to be
the representation of the fovea in striate cortex, the
center of which is marked (by me) with an X.

Thus, he thought that only subcortical lesions produced homonymous
hemianopia.[122]

Soon after these first studies by Ferrier, Hermann Munk (1839–1912),
professor of physiology at the Veterinary Hochschule in Berlin, reported very
different results on the effects of occipital lesions in dogs and monkeys,[123] and
the battle began, a battle that was not to be resolved for more than a decade.
Munk's surgical and aseptic techniques were much better than those of Ferrier,
and he was able to study his animals for many months. He described two types
of blindness after occipital lesions. The first type he called *Seelenblindheit* or
"psychic blindness," and he reported that it occurred after limited occipital
lesions in dogs. The dogs saw objects and avoided bumping into them but did
not recognize their meaning:

No abnormalities of hearing, taste, smell, motricity or sensation.
The dog walks freely about the room without bumping into
objects. If one blocks his path, he avoids or adroitly jumps over

obstacles. But within the psychic domain of vision a distinctive defect exists: he pays no attention to water or food, even if he is hungry and thirsty. He seems indifferent to everything he sees; threats do not frighten him. One can bring a match up to his eyes without him backing away. Seeing his master or seeing other dogs leaves him impassive . . . he no longer knows or recognizes what he sees.

Although these results were never replicated by others and Munk's interpretation was disputed, the term psychic blindness caught on, in part because the concept fit the associationist theories of the period.[124] Munk's observations on psychic blindness were brought to a wide audience by William James, who discussed them in detail in his *Principles of Psychology,* published in 1890. Thus, when Lissauer published the first detailed anatomic-clinical report of a human visual recognition deficit in the absence of sensory losses, he adopted Munk's term and went on to distinguish two types of psychic blindness, apperceptive and associative. Later, Sigmund Freud coined the term "visual agnosia" to replace psychic blindness.[125] However, "psychic blindness" continued to be used and was immediately applied by Heinrich Klüver and Paul Bucy to describe the behavior of their temporal-lobectomized monkeys. (See chapter 5.)

The second type of blindness Munk distinguished he called *Rindenblindheit,* or "cortical blindness." It was total absence of vision and he found that it followed complete removal of the occipital cortex in both dogs and monkeys. With his monkeys, Munk realized that complete unilateral occipital lesions produce blindness not in the opposite eye but in half of each retina. Presumably the fact that only half the retinal fibers cross in the monkey but about 80 percent of them cross in the dog made this phenomenon of homonymous hemianopsia much easier to detect by casual observation in the monkey than in the dog. As for Ferrier, Munk had this to say[126]:

In my first communication on the physiology of the cortex . . . I did not say anything about Ferrier's work on the monkey because

there was nothing good to say about it . . . [Ferrier's] statements
and what followed from them . . . are worthless and gratuitous
constructions since the operated animals were examined by Mr.
Ferrier in quite an insufficient manner . . . as the experiments show
now I have said at that time rather too little than too much, Mr.
Ferrier had not made one correct guess, all his statements have
turned out to be wrong.

About this time, Lister described his techniques for aseptic surgery, and
soon after, Ferrier and Yeo used them in a new series of cortical lesions in
monkeys.[127] Now the animals could be studied for several months after operation, and Ferrier modified his previous views as to the permanence of the
blindness after angular gyrus lesions[128]:

Formerly, I localized the visual centres in the angular gyrus, to the
exclusion of the occipital lobes. This being a partial truth is an error.
. . . Complete destruction of the angular gyri on both sides causes
for a time total blindness, succeeded by a lasting visual impairment
in both eyes. The only lesion which causes complete and permanent blindness is total destruction of the occipital lobes and angular
gyri on both sides.

Despite this retreat, Ferrier (1886) still insisted that Munk's conclusions
on the location of the visual area were "entirely erroneous" and "vitiated by
the occurrence of secondary encephalitis." Ferrier's observations on angular
gyrus lesions actually anticipated subsequent work implicating the parietal
cortex in visual functions. (See chapter 5.)

Now Edward Albert Schäfer (1850–1935), professor of physiology at
University College, London, and later at Edinburgh, entered the fray. In his
first experiments, carried out with his student Victor Horsley (coinventor of
the stereotaxic instrument), they obtained results opposite from those of Ferrier,
namely, more eye movements from stimulation of the occipital lobe than the
angular gyrus, and much greater visual deficits from occipital lesions than from

angular gyrus ones.[129] Then Schäfer carried out a series of further experiments with an American neurologist, Sanger Brown, in which the occipital lesions were more complete than anybody had made previously (figure 1.23), and they studied several of the animals in detail for several months.[130] They convincingly showed that total removal of the occipital lobe produced permanently blind animals, but only if the lesion extended on the ventral surface into the temporal lobe.

Angular gyrus involvement, however, was neither necessary nor sufficient to produce such blindness. They also failed, in several monkeys, to confirm Ferrier's claim that temporal lesions produce deafness. In explanation of this discrepancy, Schäfer suggested that Ferrier's one monkey, indisputably deaf after a temporal lesion, must have been deaf preoperatively.[131] (One of Brown and Schäfer's monkeys that retained its hearing after bilateral temporal lobectomy was a precursor to all subsequent work on the temporal lobe and vision, as discussed in chapter 5.)

Ferrier and Schäfer continued to quarrel over whether the occipital lobe or the angular gyrus was the visual area (as well as whether the temporal lobe had an auditory center), both in journals and at various national and international meetings to which they brought their critical monkeys as demonstrations and to be examined by special committees. William James in his influential *Principles of Psychology,* after complaining of all this internecine warfare, came down unambiguously for a visual area in the occipital lobes. The battle was virtually over by then.

Today, the bases for the apparent contradictions between Ferrier and Munk and Schäfer in the location of the visual area are understandable. From his descriptions and drawings (figure 1.22), it is clear that Ferrier removed the occipital lobes by an incision parallel to and about a half an inch or more posterior to the lunate sulcus. This site was chosen to make sure that the entire angular gyrus, his supposed visual center, was entirely spared. By his estimates this would remove "at least two thirds of the occipital lobes." Today we know that such a lesion would leave intact the representation of about the peripheral thirty degrees of the visual field in striate cortex and, more important, about a

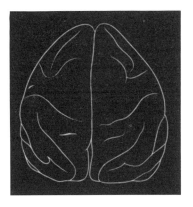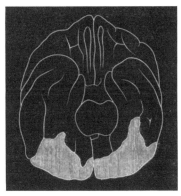

Figure 1.23   The occipital lesions that Brown and Schäfer (1888) reported to cause blindness in macaques. The lesions include what we now know to be the entire representation of the visual field in striate cortex, including both the representation of the fovea on the lateral surface (left, dorsal view) and of the extreme periphery in the far anterior of the calcarine sulcus (right, ventral view).

few degrees of the entire representation of the lower half of the vertical meridian as well.[132] This is enough residual striate cortex to account for the visually guided behavior described by Ferrier after his occipital lesions.

In contrast, Schäfer's occipital lesions included not only all the striate cortex on the lateral surface by making his lobectomy through the floor of the lunate sulcus, but in the only animal totally and permanently blind, the bilateral lesion extended on the ventral surface far enough forward to have included all the buried striate cortex in the anterior calcarine fissure. Munk provided less detailed information on the sites of his lesions, but they certainly included more of striate cortex than did Ferrier's as well as at least some of the striate cortex in the calcarine sulcus on the medial surface.

Striate Cortex Is Visual Cortex

By the turn of the century, with the resolution of the Ferrier-Schäfer-Munk debate, anatomical, clinicopathological, and experimental data were converging

73

as to the identity of the visual area in the cortex of humans and monkeys. French anatomist Gratiolet's (1854) identification of the optic radiation (initially called Gratiolet's radiation) proceeding from the geniculate to the posterior cortex was important as the first demonstration of a sensory pathway extending to the cortex. The terminus of this visual pathway was more accurately delimited in the developmental myeloarchitectonic studies of Paul Flechsig (1847–1929), professor at Leipzig, beginning in the 1870s. On the basis of the time of myelination, he divided human cortex into three zones: projection, myelinating at birth; intermediate, myelinating at one month; and terminal, myelinating later. The intermediate and terminal areas taken together he termed association cortex (figure 1.24). By 1896 Flechsig could identify the target of the visual radiations with the most posterior projection zone, and he realized it was the region of the stripe of Gennari. This region was soon named by G. Elliot Smith (1907) area striata.[133] (The concept of association cortex is discussed in chapter 5.)

During the 1880s, studies of human brain damage by Hermann Wilbrand in Hamburg, M. Allan Starr at Columbia University, Henry Hun in Albany, and others were identifying blindness with damage to the occipital cortex.[134] Swedish neuropathologist Salomon Henschen collected over 160 cases of blindness and hemianopia after cortical lesions, which led him to identify the center of vision or cortical retina with the calcarine cortex and later, with all of striate cortex. Final experimental proof of the identification of striate cortex with vision came with Minkowski's behavioral and anatomical studies in animals.[135]

The term "calcarine sulcus" was coined by T. H. Huxley (1825–1895) in the course of his bitter dispute with Richard Owen (1804–1992) over the hippocampus minor and man's place in nature. (See chapter 4.) Owen claimed that only humans had a hippocampus minor, also known as the calcar avis. This structure is a ridge in the floor of the posterior horn of the lateral ventricle. To prove Owen wrong, Huxley and his allies set out to demonstrate its existence in a variety of primates. In the course of his study of the brain of the spider monkey for this purpose, Huxley (1861) provided the first accurate description of the calcarine sulcus. He called it "calcarine" because its indentation into the lateral ventricle is what forms the calcar avis.

———

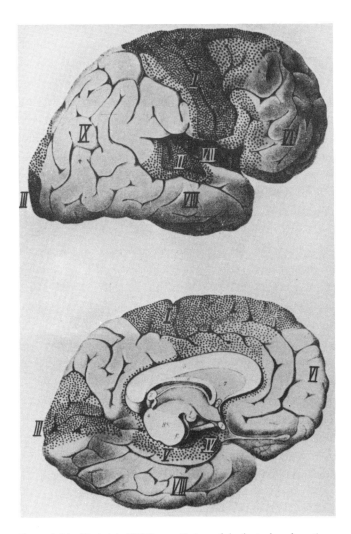

Figure 1.24 Flechsig's (1886) parcellation of the brain based on time
of myelinization. The densely stippled areas are the projection zones
surrounded by the marginal or intermediate zones. The terminal areas
are unstippled. Association cortex is made up of the intermediate and
terminal zones.

As the localization problem was being solved, the next issue was how was striate cortex was organized. The great Arab visual scientist ibn al-Haythem (965–1039), known in Europe as Alhazen, had proposed a point-to-point projection of the retinal image onto the brain.[136] This idea was well known in Europe through the translation of his work, *De Aspectibus,* the standard textbook on physiological optics until Kepler and beyond. Depictions of the visual pathways from the Renaissance onward typically show a point-to-point projection from eye to brain whether fanciful, as in Descartes (figure 1.25), or remarkably prescient, as in Newton (figure 1.20). This idea of a topographic projection seemed to have derived from the theoretical considerations of Alhazen, rather than from any empirical evidence.

Henschen, with his large number of cases, made a good start at empirically decoding the topography of striate cortex. He correctly placed the representation of the upper visual field in the lower bank of the calcarine sulcus and that of the lower one in the upper bank, but he reversed the center-periphery organization. This error was hardly surprising, given how large and diffuse many of his lesions were. As Glickstein and Whitteridge pointed out, it was the introduction of high-velocity bullets in the Russo-Japanese War that produced discrete lesions and often small entry and exit wounds, and thus made it possible to plot the locus of destroyed brain and correlate it with visual field defects. In that war, Japanese ophthalmologist Tatsuji Inouye[137] produced the first reasonably accurate scheme of how the retina is mapped on striate cortex, including magnification of the representation of the fovea, which had not been observed previously. In World War I a large number of studies reported similar results,[138] but the most widely known is that of the British neurologist Sir Gordon Holmes, perhaps because his easy-to-understand schematic diagram was reproduced in so many textbooks (figure 1.26).[139]

Neurophysiology of Striate Cortex Begins

In 1886 Adolf Beck began to work for his doctorate at the University of Kracow.[140] This was not only the period of intensive searching for sensory

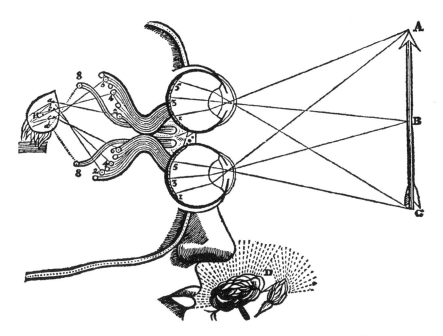

Figure 1.25   Several aspects of Descartes's theory of sensory processing are illustrated in this figure from his physiology textbook, *Treatise on Man* (1662). Light from the arrow enters the eye; the lens throws an inverted but topographically ordered image onto the retina. The message then travels in the hollow optic nerves from each eye by way of the animal spirits to the central pineal gland, where the information from the two eyes is united in a corresponding fashion to yield a single upright image. Olfactory messages from the flower also travel to the pineal body, but the strength of the visual signal (due to attention) suppresses this olfactory input.

centers in the cortex but also the beginning of electrophysiology. I. M. Sechenov and his students had recorded electrical changes in the spinal cord and brain of a frog after stimulation of its leg. Beck then set out to use this method to try to localize the different sensory systems. He wrote:

> The question arises, are there any currents in the nervous centers of the brain and spinal cord? If so, are there changes in these currents during activity? And would the localizing of such changes

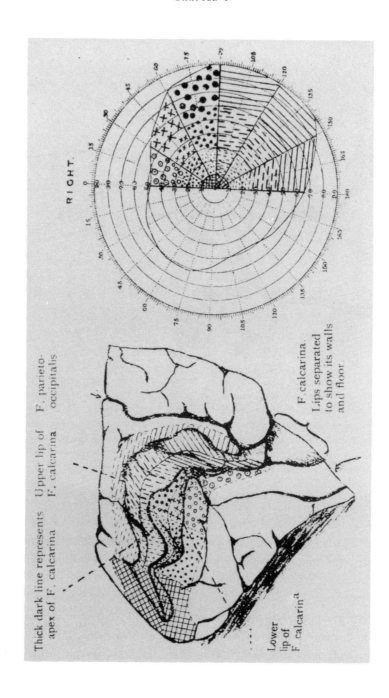

Thick dark line represents apex of F. calcarina

Upper lip of F. calcarina

F. parieto-occipitals

F. calcarina. Lips separated to show its walls and floor

Lower lip of F. calcarin[a]

be of any help in demonstrating a state of activity of a focal nature in the central nervous system?

After a series of experiments on frogs in which he thought he found spontaneous electrical activity, Beck turned to the cortex of rabbits and dogs. He placed pairs of electrodes in various cortical regions and presented visual, auditory, and tactile stimuli. He found an oscillating potential difference in the occipital region in the case of visual stimuli and used it to plot the extent of the visual cortex. As his thesis was in Polish, he published a three-page summary in German in the leading physiology journal of the day, *Centralblatt für Physiologie*. The importance of his demonstration of sensory evoked responses was immediately recognized; indeed, it stimulated a flood of letters claiming priority. One of these was from Richard Caton of Liverpool, who had published similar if less extensive experiments earlier.[141] However, not only had they gone unnoticed in Poland but they were totally ignored in England. The physiology establishment there thought Caton's "weak electric currents" quite irrelevant.

Beck went on to a distinguished academic career in Poland, including rectorship of the University of Lvov. When he was eighty, the Germans came to take him because he was a Jew. He swallowed the cyanide capsule supplied by his son, a doctor, and escaped the gas chamber.[142]

In 1934, American psychologist S. Howard Bartley was the first to carry out a systematic study of the visual evoked response of cerebral cortex and did so in rabbits. Then in the early 1940s, at Johns Hopkins, S. A. Talbot and Wade Marshall used visual evoked responses to carry out their pioneering studies of the visual topography of striate cortex first in cats, then in macaques, and then,

Figure 1.26 Representation of the retina in striate cortex according to Gordon Holmes (1918a): "A diagram of the probable representation of the different portions of the visual fields in the calcarine cortex. On the left is a drawing of the mesial surface of the left occipital lobe with the lips of the calcarine separated so that its wall and floor are visible. The markings on the various portions of the visual cortex which is thus exposed correspond with those shown in the chart of the right half of the field of vision. This diagram does not claim to be in any respect accurate; it is merely a scheme."

with Clinton Woolsey and others, in a variety of other mammals. Particularly in gyrocephalic animals, these maps tended to be incomplete, since the macroelectrodes used confined the recordings to the surface of the cortex. Subsequently, as described in the next section, using single-neuron recording, Daniel and Whitteridge in the monkey and Hubel and Wiesel in the cat, followed by many other studies, confirmed and extended these electrophysiological maps of the visuotopic organization of striate cortex.[143]

The Microelectrode Arrives; from Adrian to Kuffler

The analysis of visual processing by single neurons begins with the work of E. A. Adrian. Indeed, virtually all of modern neurophysiology begins with Adrian. Among his other achievements were the establishment of the all-or-none law, the first recording from single neurons, the concepts of labeled line and rate coding, the first recording of spontaneous activity from cerebral and cerebellar cortex neurons, and confirmation of the existence of brain waves, the electroencephalogram.[144] Titles and awards accrued: he was made a baron, was awarded the Order of Merit and the Nobel prize (1932), and was elected master of Trinity College and professor of physiology in the University of Cambridge, and president of the Royal Society and of the British Association for the Advancement of Science.

In 1927 he and Bryan Matthews recorded spike trains from the optic nerve of the conger eel and noted that the rate of firing increased and the latency decreased as the intensity of the light increased. Following this up, H. Keffer Hartline dissected out single optic fibers first in *Limulus,* the horseshoe crab, and then in the frog, where he distinguished on, off, and on-off responses for the first time and introduced the concept of a visual receptive field.[145] Hartline spent most of his career at the University of Pennsylvania and Rockefeller University, and shared the Nobel prize with George Wald and Ragnar Granit in 1967.

The next major development was that of Stephen Kuffler, then at the John Hopkins University. Working with cats, he developed a technique for recording from the retina without having to remove the cornea and lens, as had been done previously. This maintained the normal optics of the eye and enabled him to focus light on the portion of the retina that he was recording from. With these techniques he discovered the center-surround, on-off antagonistic organization of the receptive fields of retinal ganglion cells.[146] Horace Barlow, who was working in Kuffler's laboratory, had made similar observations in the frog earlier. He noted that this receptive field organization made the cells much more sensitive to edges and contours than to diffuse light. (Barlow even called one of the class of cells he described a bug detector.) We now know that this receptive field structure is fundamental to the organization of the entire visual system. It was the extension of Kuffler's work from retina to cortex by Hubel and Wiesel that formed the basis of current study of visual cortex.

Hubel and Wiesel

In 1959, two physicians, David Hubel, a Canadian, and Torsten Wiesel, a Swede, came to Kuffler's laboratory in Baltimore as postdoctoral fellows. Visual physiology, and indeed all of sensory physiology and psychology, were never the same again. Through the brilliant use of single-neuron physiology they revealed the functional architecture of striate cortex. This research promised the possibility of understanding perception in terms of neurons, and became the model for subsequent explorations of visual neurons inside and outside of striate cortex and for all of contemporary neurophysiology. Subsequently, Hubel and Wiesel moved to Harvard with Kuffler, and in 1981 they shared the Nobel prize with Roger Sperry. Their remarkable achievements that extended into visual neuroanatomy and neural development have been widely reviewed and will not concern us here except for two historical notes.[147]

The first is the description of their first observation of an orientation selective neuron in a cat, perhaps the opening wedge in revealing the secrets of striate cortex[148]:

We had been doing experiments for about a month . . . and were not getting very far; the cells simply would not respond to our spots and annuli. [The stimuli that had been used by Kuffler to reveal the properties of retinal ganglion cells.] One day we made an especially stable recording. . . . For 3 or 4 hours we got absolutely nowhere. Then gradually we began to elicit some vague and inconsistent responses by stimulating somewhere in the mid-periphery of the retina. We were inserting [a] glass slide with a black spot into a [projecting ophthalmoscope] when suddenly over the audiomonitor the cell went off like a machine gun. After some fussing and fiddling we found out what was happening. The response had nothing to do with the black dot. As the glass slide was inserted its edge was casting onto the retina a faint but sharp shadow, a straight dark line on a light background. That was what the cell wanted, and it wanted it, moreover, in just one narrow range of orientations.

A few years later they realized that cells with similar orientation selectivity and cells with similar ocular dominance were arranged in orientation and ocular dominance columns, respectively. This discovery must have been facilitated by the proximity at Hopkins of Vernon Mountcastle, who had recently discovered columnar organization in somatosensory cortex.[149]

The second historical point is that Hubel and Wiesel were by no means the first to record from single neurons in striate cortex. In 1952 the Freiburg group starring R. Jung, G. Baumgartener, O. Creutzfeldt, and O. J. Grusser had begun a systematic program of research on the visual activity of single neurons in striate cortex of the cat.[150] Although their techniques were technically sophisticated, their central finding for about the first ten years was actually that striate neurons showed little visual responsiveness: 50 percent of the many cells sampled showed no responses, and the responses of many of the others, by subsequent standards, were rather feeble. As Jung later candidly admitted, a primary reason for their failure to activate striate cells was that their elaborate apparatus (which took two years to build) was too inflexible to vary the orientation of the visual stimulus. As he put it, "We missed the orientation specificity . . . [because of] . . . premature quantification and a too rigid methodological restriction."[151]

———

This completes our story of research on striate cortex. The discovery and study of visual areas outside striate cortex is recounted in chapter 5.

NOTES

1. Breasted, 1930. The village was probably Qurna, which was recently bulldozed by the Egyptian government. *New York Times,* March 4, 1997.

2. Sarton, 1959; Sigerist, 1951.

3. Breasted, 1930.

4. Breasted, 1930.

5. Hurray, 1928; Sigerist, 1951; Guthrie, 1945.

6. Sarton, 1959; Sigerist, 1951.

7. Breasted, 1930.

8. Sarton, 1959; Sigerist, 1951.

9. Herodotus, 1910.

10. Sarton, 1959; Sigerist, 1951.

11. Keele, 1957.

12. Keele, 1957.

13. Zimmer, 1948. Or was the chief being metaphorical or perhaps sarcastic?

14. As in *The Yellow Emperor's Classic,* compiled from earlier sources in the third century BCE (Huang Ti, 1949; Porkert, 1974). On the other hand, in vol. 5, pt. 5 of his monumental *Science and Civilization in China,* Joseph Needham (1983) tells us ". . . the brain was always an organ of cardinal importance in Taoist anatomy and physiology," which he footnotes thus: "Exactly what its functions were considered to be is not so easy to say. We shall return to all these matters in sect. 43 on physiology in Vol. 6 . . ." Needham died in 1995 as vol. 6, pt. 3 containing sect. 42 went to press. Whether his successors will fulfill his promise to discuss the importance of the brain remains to be seen. The brain is mentioned often in the context of Taoist sexual techniques (Needham, 1983; Chang, 1977; Van Gulik, 1961; Ware, 1966). Withholding ejaculation was thought to enable the semen to be rerouted up the spinal cord to "nourish" and "repair" the brain. (The Taoist adept apparently could achieve orgasm without ejaculation.) Conserving semen was believed to lead to long life or even immortality, as in this Taoist saying provided by Needham (1983):

> who wishes life unending to attain
> must raise the essence to restore the brain.

———

15. Spence, 1985.

16. All the works of the presocratic philosopher-scientists are lost. All we have are quotations or fragments collected by the ancient doxographers. These were assembled by H. Diels at the beginning of the century and translated into English by Freeman (1954). This account depends on her translations, Schrodinger's (1954) appreciation, and the works of Sarton (1959), Sigerist (1961) Longrigg (1993), Farrington (1944), and others cited below.

17. Freeman, 1954; Sarton, 1959; Lloyd, 1970.

18. Farrington, 1944.

19. Lloyd, 1975; Edelstein, 1967a; Longrigg, 1993; Theophrastus, 1917.

20. Grusser and Hagner, 1990.

21. Theophrastus, 1917; Freeman, 1954; Beare, 1906.

22. Singer, 1957; Galen, 1968.

23. Freeman, 1954; Beare, 1906.

24. Smith, 1979; Lloyd, 1978.

25. Hippocrates, 1950.

26. Edelstein, 1967b.

27. The standard convention for citing Plato is the pagination used in the first Greek-Latin edition published by Henricus Stephanus (1578).

28. Lloyd, 1970; Sarton, 1959; and Farrington, 1949, respectively.

29. Sarton, 1959; Needham, 1959; Mayr, 1982; Nordenskiold, 1928. On the other hand, for ridicule by a nobelist, see Medawar and Medawar (1983).

30. Grene, 1963; Gotthelf and Lennox, 1987; Devereux and Pellegrin, 1990.

31. Sarton, 1959; Longrigg, 1993.

32. Galen, 1962, 1968.

33. Aristotle's works here, and generally, are cited by the page numbers given by I. Bekker in the nineteenth century. The abbreviations for individual works used here are GA, *Generation of Animals;* HA, *History of Animals;* PA, *Parts of Animals;* SS, "On Sense and Sensible Objects" in *Parva Naturalia;* SW, "On Sleep and Waking" in *Parva Naturalia;* and YO, "On Youth and Old Age" in *Parva Naturalia.*

34. Lones, 1912.

35. Clarke, 1963; Clarke and Stannard, 1963.

36. Avicenna, 1930.

37. Schlomoh, 1953.

38. Through Sir Richard Burton, 1885.

39. Lloyd, 1975.

———

40. Praxagoras's fragments were collected and translated by Steckerl (1958).

41. Farrington, 1949; Fraser, 1972.

42. Longrigg, 1993; Canfora, 1990.

43. Canfora, 1990.

44. Von Staden, 1989; Dobson, 1926–1927; Longrigg, 1988. Von Staden (1989) collected and translated the fragments of Herophilus, and Dobson (1926–1927) those of Erasistratus.

45. Fraser, 1972; Von Staden, 1989; Longrigg, 1988; Edelstein, 1967b.

46. Fraser, 1972.

47. Fraser, 1972.

48. Longrigg, 1988.

49. For German human vivisection see Lifton (1986); for Japanese see Harris (1994); for the revival of human dissection, Singer (1957).

50. Von Staden, 1989; Dobson, 1926–1927; Longrigg, 1988.

51. Galen, 1968.

52. Schiller, 1965; Clarke and Dewhurst, 1996.

53. Galen, 1968.

54. Lloyd, 1973.

55. Von Staden, 1989; Longrigg, 1988, 1993.

56. Sarton, 1954; Siegel, 1968, 1970; Lloyd, 1973.

57. Galen, 1968, 1956, 1962, and 1978–1984, respectively. Each of these relatively recent translations is the first into English. Many other works remain untranslated into English.

58. Woolam, 1958; Spillane, 1981.

59. Pagel, 1958; Clarke, 1962; Woolam, 1957.

60. Lewy, 1847.

61. Nemesius, 1955.

62. Corner, 1927.

63. Hunter and Macalpine, 1963.

64. From the Renaissance until well into the eighteenth century, Padua was by far the principal medical school accessible to Jewish students from all of Europe. Between 1617 and 1816 alone at least 350 received joint doctoral degrees in medicine and philosophy and many more attended without matriculating (Ruderman, 1995). Many of them arrived with little knowledge of Latin, Italian, or any aspect of life and culture outside of the shtetels and ghettos. The Jewish community in Padua provided boarding schools to prepare such students for entrance to the medical school while enveloping them in a Jewish support network.

65. Oporinus had been a medical secretary to Paracelsus, "the Dr. Faustus of the sixteenth century," and Professor of Greek and Latin at the University of Basel before turning to printing only a year before he published Vesalius (Le Roy Ladurie, 1997). Later he published the first Latin edition of the Koran, which got him jailed. He was released with the help of Martin Luther (Saunders and O'Malley, 1950).

66. Singer, 1952.

67. Singer, 1952.

68. Singer, 1952.

69. Meyer, 1971; Clarke and O'Malley, 1996.

70. Meyer, 1971; Clarke and O'Malley, 1996.

71. Nordenskiold, 1928.

72. Clarke and Bearn, 1968.

73. Meyer, 1971.

74. Clarke and O'Malley, 1996.

75. Bartholin, 1656 quoted in Schiller, 1965; Meyer, 1971.

76. Dow, 1940; Dewhurst, 1982; Meyer and Hierons, 1965.

77. Willis, 1664.

78. Willis, 1664.

79. Neuburger, 1981; Kruger, 1963.

80. Neuburger, 1981.

81. Neuburger, 1981.

82. Gennari, 1782, quoted in Fulton, 1937.

83. Neuburger, 1981.

84. Gennari, 1782, quoted in Fulton, 1937.

85. Although he never held an academic post, Vicq d'Azyr (1748–1794) was renowned as an anatomist (the mammillothalamic tract bears his name) and as a physician, Marie Antoinette being one of his more famous patients.

86. Glickstein and Rizzolatti, 1984.

87. Clarke and O'Malley, 1996.

88. Glickstein and Rizzolatti, 1984.

89. Gall preferred the term "organology" over Spurzheim's "phrenology." For differences between the more cautious Gall and the more popularizing Spurzheim, see Clarke and Jacyna (1987) and Zola-Morgan (1995).

90. Temkin, 1953.

91. Gall and Spurzheim, 1835.

———

92. Gross, 1987a; Young, 1970b.

93. Cooter, 1985.

94. Young, 1970b; Clarke and Jacyna, 1987; Clarke and O'Malley, 1996.

95. Carpenter, 1845.

96. Meyer, 1971.

97. Young, 1970b; Clarke and Jacyna, 1987; Broca, 1861.

98. Bouillard was known as the "red dean" for his participation in the Revolution of 1848. He reportedly prided himself on being the model for Balzac's Dr. Horace Bianchon (Schiller, 1979).

99. Young, 1970b; Clarke and Jacyna, 1987; Broca, 1861.

100. Young, 1970b; Boakes, 1984.

101. Hofstadter, 1955.

102. Hofstadter, 1955.

103. Spencer, 1855.

104. Jackson, 1958; Young, 1970b.

105. Fritsch and Hitzig, 1870.

106. Müller, 1838.

107. This is an example of an intromission theory of vision. Extromission holds that something streams out of the eye and interacts with the seen object (e.g., Euclid). More complicated interactive formulations (e.g., Aristotle) were also held among the Greek visual scientist-philosophers (Theophrastus, 1917; Lindberg 1976). Today, most children and many adults still hold extromission views of vision (Winer and Cottrell, 1966).

108. Von Helmholtz, 1863.

109. In 1845 Von Helmholtz, du Bois-Reymond, and two other students of Müller, Carl Ludwig and Ernst Brucke (Freud's teacher), all of whom later became famous as founders of modern physiology, got together to issue a manifesto against vitalism, the doctrine that life cannot be reduced to physics and chemistry. Perhaps not coincidentally, Müller was the last great (mainstream) biologist who was a vitalist. Their manifesto declared, "No other forces than common physical chemical ones are active within the organism," and they proceeded to support this reductionism in every branch of physiology (Coleman, 1971, particularly, the bibliography; Boring, 1950).

110. Boring, 1950; cf. Sur et al., 1988.

111. Bell's (1811) account, was in a "tiny little" pamphlet of thirty-six pages, each with 4.5 × 2.5 inches of text per page, entitled *Idea of a New Anatomy of the Brain,* 100 copies of which were privately printed for his friends. It did not seem to be noticed in Europe, although it

───────

was published in toto in an American medical journal at the time (Bell, 1812). A long and bitter priority controversy arose between Bell and the great French physiologist Francois Magendie (1783–1855) over the discovery of the law of spinal roots (i.e., that ventral spinal roots are motor and dorsal ones sensory). In fact, (a) Bell proposed only the sensory functions of the dorsal roots, (b) there is no reason to believe that Magendie knew of Bell's claims before he carried out and published his own experiments, and (c) both halves of the law were experimentally demonstrated by Magendie, whereas Bell's consideration of the functions of the dorsal roots were largely anatomically based. See Cranefield, 1974.

112. Bell, 1811.

113. Gall and Spurzheim, 1835.

114. Panizza, 1855; Mazzarello and Della Sala, 1993.

115. Carpenter, 1845; Walshe, 1958.

116. Tamburini, 1880; Manni and Petrosini, 1994. A parallel to the neglect of Panizza's work because it was ahead of its time was the fate of Gregor Mendel's (1866) paper on inheritance in peas, which although published in an equally obscure journal, also passed into the major libraries and across the desks of the biology savants of the day, to whom it apparently had no meaning. The difference was that when Tamburini (1880) rediscovered Panizza, Munk had already gone beyond him. In contrast, when Mendel was rediscovered by De Vries in about 1900, Mendel's work was still original and important (Mayr, 1982).

117. Ferrier, 1873, 1875a. In the beginning Ferrier was very stingy in giving Fritsch and Hitzig credit for their methods and discoveries. Thus, when he submitted his paper (Ferrier, 1875b) to the prestigious *Philosophical Transactions of the Royal Society,* one of the referees, Michael Foster, objected to his failure to credit adequately Fritsch and Hitzig. T. H. Huxley was then called in as a third referee "for the purpose of ascertaining . . . whether Dr. Ferrier has or has not done sufficient justice to the labors of his predecessors" (Royal Society archives, RR.7.302). Ferrier added a more explicit recognition of their priority, but the referees still were not satisfied. In the end, Ferrier refused to make enough of the requested changes and preferred to omit all his experiments on dogs, only the ones on monkeys (which Fritsch and Hitzig had not used) making it into print (the referee reports and Ferrier's replies are in the Royal Society archives, RR.7.299–305 and MC.10.194; see also Young, 1970b).

118. Ferrier, 1875b, 1876.

119. Ferrier, 1878.

120. Newton, 1952.

121. Polyak, 1957.

122. Ferrier, 1878.

123. Munk, 1881. The passage quoted was translated by Hécaen and Albert, 1978.

124. Hécaen and Albert, 1978; James, 1890.

125. James, 1890; Lissauer, 1890; Freud, 1891.

126. Munk, 1881.

127. Ferrier and Yeo, 1884, Ferrier, 1886.

128. Ferrier and Yeo, 1884; Ferrier, 1886.

129. Horsley and Schäfer, 1888. Later, Schäfer changed his name to Sharpey-Schäfer to "emphasise his veneration" for William Sharpey, his mentor and predecessor in the University College chair (Sherrington, 1935; Marshall, 1949). Both Horsley and his mentor Schäfer were strong advocates of women's rights, and Horsley was also a militant temperance crusader, particularly against the traditional alcohol ration given to British soldiers and sailors, even when brain injured. Perhaps because of his strong advocacy of unpopular views, Horsley, although a distinguished neurosurgeon, was sent to the Middle East campaign in World War I rather than to a rear-guard hospital. He died of a fever there (Lyons, 1966; Paget, 1949). Schäfer, Horsley, and Ferrier were all knighted for their work in physiology and medicine in that very British manner of carefully rewarding the worthy, even foreign-born like Schäfer and troublemakers like Horsley.

130. Brown and Schäfer, 1888; Schäfer, 1888a, b.

131. Ferrier, 1888, Schäfer 1888a, b, 1990.

132. Gattass et al., 1981.

133. Gratiolet, 1854; Flechsig, 1886; Elliot Smith, 1907.

134. Polyak, 1957.

135. Henschen, 1893; Minkowski, 1911.

136. Gross, 1981; Lindberg, 1976.

137. Glickstein and Whitteridge, 1987; Inouye, 1909; Holmes, 1918a.

138. Polyak, 1957.

139. Glickstein and Whitteridge, 1987; Inouye, 1909; Holmes, 1918a.

140. Brazier, 1988.

141. Beck, 1890, 1973; Caton, 1875.

142. Brazier, 1988.

143. Bartley, 1934; Talbot and Marshall, 1941; Woolsey, 1971; Daniel and Whitteridge, 1961; Hubel and Weisel, 1962.

144. Adrian, 1928, 1947.

145. Adrian and Matthews, 1927; Hartline and Graham, 1932; Hartline, 1938.
146. Kuffler, 1953; Barlow, 1953.
147. Hubel and Wiesel, 1959, 1962; Hubel, 1988.
148. Hubel, 1982.
149. Hubel and Wiesel, 1962; Mountcastle, 1957.
150. Jung, 1992.
151. Jung, 1992.

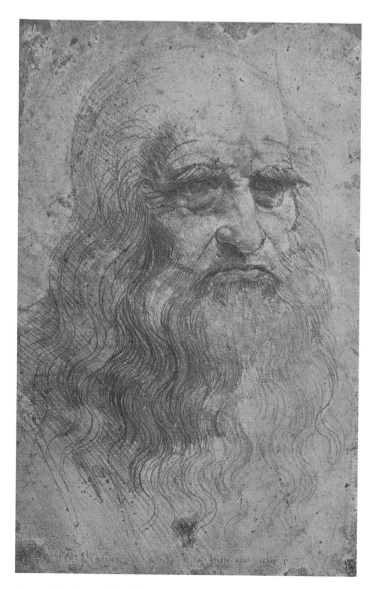

Figure 2.1   Leonardo's self-portrait (?), ca. 1510–1513. Turin, Royal Library.

Leonardo da Vinci's powerful, insatiable, and extraordinarily visual curiosity drove him to seek meaning in both the structure and pattern of the microcosm of the body and the macrocosm of the universe.[1] For him, to draw was to understand. Throughout most of his life he had a consuming interest in the structure and function of the eye, brain, and nervous system, and in a variety of visual phenomena such as illusions, contrast, and color.[2–6] Although he was initially led to these subjects by his painting or, as he put it, "the science of painting," they soon became obsessions in their own right.

Leonardo (1452–1519) was the first great medical illustrator.[7–10] His are the earliest surviving naturalistic drawings of the internal structure of the human body. Furthermore, he introduced a number of powerful techniques for portraying anatomical structures such as the use of transparencies, cross sections, exploded figures, and three-dimensional shading.[11] Today, his anatomical drawings continue to attract huge crowds, although most are unaware of the frequent errors they contain and their dependence on traditional authority.

This chapter concerns Leonardo's drawings of the nervous system. First, I consider the background of neuroanatomy in fifteenth-century Europe, then the development of some of Leonardo's ideas on the brain and the eye, and finally, the impact of this work. Leonardo may be the paradigmatic Renaissance genius with ideas about such things as airplanes, submarines, machine guns, and bicycles that were not to be realized until the twentieth century. However, in his neuroscience he begins solidly in the Middle Ages, blinded, or at least blinkered, by traditional dogma. Only gradually, and only partially, does he free himself from a "debased medieval Aristotelianism and a corrupted Galenism"[12] and begin to draw with accuracy the open body before him.

NEUROANATOMY IN THE FIFTEENTH CENTURY

After the death of Galen in 199, anatomical dissection for either scientific or medical reasons was absent in both Europe and Islam for over a thousand years. It began again in thirteenth-century Italy, first for forensic purposes and then as a way of illustrating Galen's anatomical works for medical students.[17] Galen, however, did not become available in direct translation until the sixteenth century; before then his work was presented by Avicenna and other Arab scientists who never practiced dissection themselves. Not only were the accounts of Galen's work indirect, but Galen never mentioned that his anatomical descriptions were almost always based on nonhumans, a fact that was not realized until recently. Galen's anatomy is remarkably accurate when applied to the monkey or ox, his usual subjects, but not to humans.[18, 19]

Box 2.1   Leonardo's Drawings and Notes

> Over 5,000 sheets of drawings and notes by Leonardo on a fantastic range of subjects have survived and are scattered in libraries around the world. In spite of his plans for a number of books, including one on anatomy, none of his drawings or texts were published until long after his death. By 1690 virtually all of his extant anatomical drawings found their way to the Royal Library in Windsor Castle, including the originals of figures 2.2, 2.3, 2.4, 2.6, 2.7, and 2.8. They are here referred to by the numbers assigned by Clark,[13] e.g., W19097. Leonardo's surviving texts, except for the recently discovered Madrid codices,[14] have been translated into English and arranged by Richter[15] and, easier to use, MacCurdy.[16]

The first European anatomy textbook was the forty-page *Anothomia* of Mondino de' Luzzi (Mundinus) written in 1316. It was essentially a dissection guide for learning Arab accounts of Galen's words, not for learning about the actual body. Mondino's work went through many manuscript editions before it was finally printed in 1478, but remained unillustrated until an edition of 1521.[20–22] It was known to Leonardo at the beginning of his dissections (around 1490) and was an important source of anatomical nomenclature for him.[23–26] An earlier medieval tradition of drawing diagrams of the human body in a froglike posture was used to represent the major organs or venisection sites. However, none of the extant ones were drawn from actual dissections, but are symbolic representations of general Greek or Arab ideas about the body, its diseases, and their treatment.[27–29]

Accurate illustrations of the body beneath the skin began not in medical schools but in the workshops of Renaissance artists. With the growth of naturalism, artists desired more accurate knowledge of the surface musculature and used the scalpel on human cadavers to obtain it. Furthermore, there seems to have been considerable interaction between Italian Renaissance artists and medical workers. Both physicians and painters belonged to and were regulated by the Guild of Physicians and Apothecaries, as was the case for surgeons, undertakers, distillers, booksellers, and silk merchants. Painters bought their pigments at the same shops where doctors bought their medicines, and human dissections were usually open to the public.[30–33]

Among the early artists who dissected human bodies to gain a more accurate view of the superficial muscles were Leonardo's teacher Verrocchio, who worked on a sculpture of the satyr Marsyas who was flayed alive for his overambition, and Verrocchio's neighbor Antoni Pollaiuolo, who displayed his anatomical knowledge particularly in his Martyrdom of St. Sebastian. Later, Michelangelo, Raphael, and Dürer all left drawings of their dissections; Dürer actually "appropriated" some of Leonardo's anatomical drawings. Leonardo's interest in anatomy presumably also began as an aid to painting, but he alone among Renaissance artists went far deeper than the appearance of the surface musculature.[34–39]

———

SEXUAL INTERCOURSE

One of Leonardo's earliest anatomical drawings (ca. 1493) and one of the first to be published, in 1795, depicted sexual intercourse (figure 2.2).[40, 41] It is headed, "I display to men the origin of their . . . cause of existence,"[42] and consists of a contradictory collection of traditional views quite unencumbered by actual observations. Avicenna believed that semen, carrying the soul of the future person, came from the spinal cord, a view he presumably obtained from the Hippocratic work *On Generation*. The idea that semen derives from the brain and travels down the spinal cord is also found in Alcmaeon and other presocratic natural philosophers.[43] To accommodate this view, Leonardo drew a hollow nerve from the spinal cord to the upper of two canals in the penis. In contrast, Galen[44] argued that sperm came from the testes; to accommodate that view, Leonardo drew a tube from the testes to the lower canal, which was thought to be used for the passage of urine as well as semen. The two canals are shown more clearly in the two drawings in the bottom left.

Both the cervix and the uterus are shown expanded, following Avicenna, who believed both structures opened up during intercourse. Note the large sperm entering the (penislike?) open cervix. There is a nerve from the uterus to the breast, illustrating the belief that in pregnancy the "retained menses" is carried to the breast and there stimulates the formation of milk. Another nerve runs from the testes to the heart, following Aristotle's theory of the heart as the center of sensation, a view subsequently abandoned by Leonardo and never held by Galen or most classical physician–philosophers.[45]

This early drawing is typical in that it serves both as an uncritical "review of the literature" and as a program for investigation. Thus, Leonardo wrote beside the drawing:

> Note what the testicles have to do with coition and the sperm. And how the foetus breathes and how it is nourished by the umbilical cord, and why one soul governs two bodies . . . and why a child of eight months does not live. . . . How the testicles are the source of ardor.

———

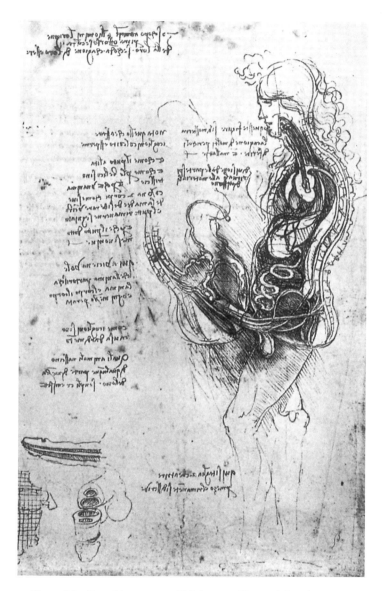

Figure 2.2   Sexual intercourse. This is one of Leonardo's earliest anatomical drawings and is particularly replete with errors (ca. 1493) W19097. (See boxes 2.1 and 2.2).

And he criticized Avicenna:

> Here Avicenna pretends that the soul generates the soul and the body the body and every member in error.

Syphilis had become widespread in Italy about this time, and at the bottom of the page Leonardo noted: "Through these figures will be demonstrated the cause of many dangers of ulcers and diseases." He returned to the subject in subsequent scattered notes. On sexual intercourse he wrote:

> The act of coitus and the parts employed therein are so repulsive that if it were not for the beauty of the faces and the adornments of the actions and the frantic state of mind, nature would lose the human species. (W19009r) . . . The woman commonly has a desire quite the opposite of that of a man. That is, the woman likes the size of the genital member of the man to be as large as possible, and the man desires the opposite in the genital member of the woman, so that neither one nor the other ever attains his interest because Nature, who cannot be blamed, has so provided because of parturition. (W19101r)

He did answer his question on the role of the "testicles in ardour"[46]:

> Testicles . . . contain in themselves ardour, that is, they are the augmenters of the animosity and ferocity of the animals; and experience shows us this clearly in the castrated animals, of which one sees the bull, the boar, the ram and the cock, very fierce animals, which after having been deprived of these testicles remain very cowardly.

Leonardo was the first to realize that in erection, the penis fills with blood.[47] On the subject of the penis he notes that it[48]:

Box 2.2   Leonardo's Handwriting

Leonardo's mirror writing is very hard to decipher and not only because it is mirror writing. He had his own peculiar orthography that changed over time, he arbitrarily fused and divided words, he used no punctuation, and he had his own set of abbreviations and symbols.[49] The mirror writing presumably reflected that he was left-handed and had been taught as a child to write with his right hand rather than any "secret code."[50] He did protect many of his inventions by introducing an intentional error into his plans such as an extra cogwheel.[51, 52]

. . . confers with the human intelligence and sometimes has intelligence of itself, and although the will of man desires to stimulate it, it remains obstinate and takes its own course, and moving sometimes of itself without license or thought by the man, whether he be sleeping or waking, and many times the man is awake and it is asleep, and many times the man wishes it to practice and it does not wish it; many times it wishes it and the man forbids it. It seems therefore that this creature has often a life and intelligence separate from the man and it would appear that the man is in the wrong in being ashamed to give it a name or exhibit it . . .

AN EARLY FIGURE SHOWING THE VENTRICULAR THEORY

As in other areas of his investigations, Leonardo's understanding of the brain shows progression over the years. He begins with uncritical notes from contemporary sources and, finding them unsatisfactory, moves on to critical inquiry and then, sometimes, to new insights.

Another one of Leonardo's earliest anatomical drawings shows the visual input to the brain (figure 2.3) It is a curious and uncritical amalgam of Arabic and medieval sources, with a minor discovery and some new techniques thrown in.[53-56] The terms for the layers from hair to brain are from Avicenna through Mondino's text; in two cases the Arabic terms are still in use today—dura mater

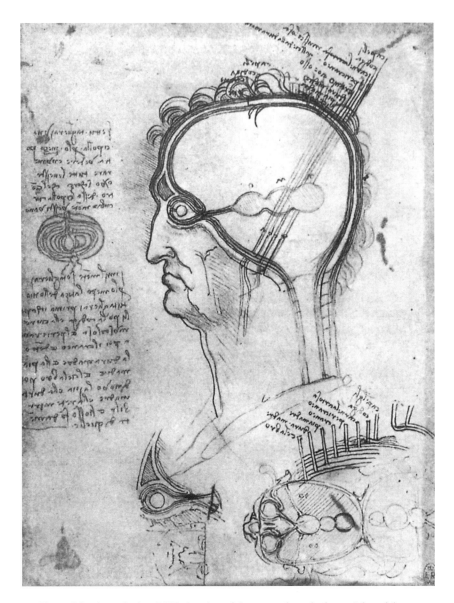

Figure 2.3   An early (ca. 1490) drawing of the eye and cerebral ventricles of the brain that uncritically combines Greek, Arab, and medieval views. W12603r

and pia mater. The depictions of the dura and pia extending to sheath the optic nerve and the eyeball (center and lower right) are again derived from Avicenna. The lens or crystalline humor is shown central, as it is in virtually all Arab and European drawings until Felix Platter (1603), the first to understand its role as a lens projecting the image onto a sensitive retina.[57, 58] The lens is shown as round, although Galen and most of the Arab authorities on the eye, but not many medieval writers, had described it more correctly.[59, 60]

Leonardo must have been uncertain about the shape of the crystalline humor, because later, in his unpublished monograph on vision,[61] he suggested and diagrammed a method for determining the shape and location of the lens:

> In the anatomy of the eye in order to see the inside well without spilling its humour one should place the whole eye in white of egg, make it boil, and become solid, cutting the egg and the eye transversely in order that none of the middle portion may be poured out.

He never carried out this idea, as reflected in his continuing to draw the crystalline humor (lens) round and his reminder to himself to "study the anatomy of different eyes."[62]

The portrayal of the ventricles as three connected spheres is not derived from Avicenna or Galen, or any other classical text. Galen knew that the first or lateral ventricles are paired, and he provided an accurate account of the morphology of all four cerebral ventricles on the basis of his dissections of the ox.[63, 64] Rather than following Galen, Leonardo depicted three circular ventricles according to the widespread medieval theory of the ventricular localization of psychological function. In the basic form of the theory, the faculties of the mind (derived from Aristotle) were distributed among the spaces within the brain (derived from those described by Galen). The lateral ventricles were collapsed into one space, the first cell or small room. This received input from all the sense organs and was the site of the sensus communis, or common sense, which integrated across the modalities. The sensations yielded images, and thus, the first cell was the seat of fantasy and imagination as well. The second or middle cell was the site of cognitive processes, reasoning, judgment, and thought. The third cell or ventricle was the site of memory. (For a discussion of the origins, variations, and longevity of the ventricular doctrine, see chapter 1 and figure 1.7.)

In the bottom figure Leonardo reflects the standard medieval concept of the location of common sense in the first ventricle by showing input to it from the eyes and ears. Note the absence of the optic chiasm, although it had been noted by Aristotle, discussed in detail by Galen, and diagrammed repeatedly in the Arab literature, including in Alhazen's *De Aspectibus,* which was the standard textbook on optics in Europe until Kepler in the sixteenth century (see figure 1.6).[65–68]

The new and correct anatomical feature, if somewhat exaggerated, is the frontal sinus, shown above the eye in the central and lower left figures. The three ways of labeling the layers of the scalp and the "unhinging" of the skull in the lower right drawing are apparently new illustration techniques.

Injecting Wax to Reveal the Ventricles

A few years later, Leonardo returned to the ventricles with brilliant success, using the sculptural technique of wax injection to reveal their shape (figure 2.4). As he instructed[69]:

> Make two vent-holes in the horns of the great ventricles, and insert melted wax with a syringe, making a hole in the ventricle of the memoria and through such a hole fill the three ventricles of the brain. Then, when the wax has set, take away the brain and you will see the shape of the ventricles. But first put narrow tubes into the vents so that the air which is in these ventricles can escape and make room for the wax which enters into the ventricles.

The shortcomings of his wax cast of the lateral ventricles seen in figure 2.4 were probably due to the absence of air vents in the posterior horns and

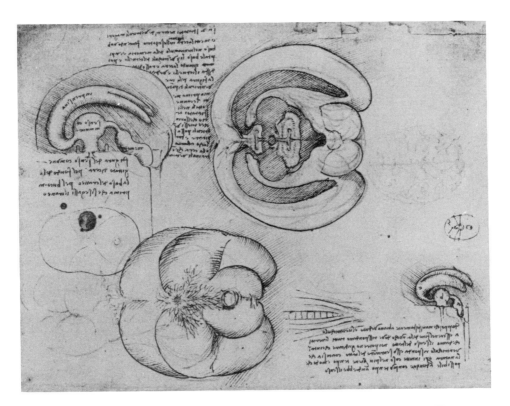

Figure 2.4   The ventricles based on wax injection and (lower) the rete mirable, ca. 1504–1507.
W19127r

the use of an unpreserved brain. This method for revealing the shape of internal
biological cavities was not used again until Frederick Ruysch in the eighteenth
century, an achievement the French Academy of Science thought equal to
Newton's.[70]

The ventral view shows a rete mirabile, a vascular structure found in the
ox, where Galen described it, but not in humans. The sulcal pattern is also that
of an ox, whereas the location of the cerebellum and the form of the ventricles
are closer to that of a human brain. Perhaps Leonardo injected both species and
this is a composite figure.[71]

As Leonardo began to study the brain itself, his attribution of functions to the ventricles became somewhat contradictory and was eventually abandoned. In the period of this drawing, he had been dissecting the cranial nerves and observed that the trigeminal and auditory nerves entered the central portion of the brain rather than the anterior portion. Therefore, in contrast to tradition and his previous drawing (figure 2.3), he put the common sense in the middle ventricle, now the third ventricle since the anterior ventricle was paired. The auditory and trigeminal inputs to the middle ventricle are diagrammed in the small horizontal section in the middle right of figure 2.5. The visual input still went to the first ventricle before proceeding to the common sense. Now he put intellect and *imprensiva* into the first ventricle. Leonardo's placement of intellect at the target of the optic nerves underlies the dominant role he gave to this sense. By "imprensiva," a term never used before or after Leonardo, he meant something like sensory processing or sensation. Although the imprensiva is never described as only visual, note that in this figure it receives only visual input. Leonardo again contradicts his idea that it initially processes all the senses by having the tactile input come to the fourth ventricle:

> Since we have clearly seen that the fourth ventricle is at the end of the medulla where all the nerves which provide the sense of touch come together, we can conclude that the sense of touch passes to this ventricle. (W19127r)

He never resolved these tensions between his anatomy and his functional localizations, and there is little effort to relate the sensory input to the ventricles in later drawings (e.g., figures 2.4 and 2.5). He did return to the medulla in the only experiment that he is known to have carried out on a living animal (he was an antivivisectionist and a vegetarian[72, 73]):

> The frog suddenly dies when its spinal medulla is perforated. . . .
> It seems therefore that here lies the foundations of motion and life.
> (W12613v)

Box 2.3   Leonardo on the Role of Anatomical Illustrations

"Dispel from your mind the thought that an understanding of the human body in every aspect of its structure can be given in words; for the more thoroughly you describe, the more you will confuse the mind of the reader and the more you will prevent him from a knowledge of the thing described; it is therefore necessary to draw as well as describe . . . I advise you not to trouble with words unless you are speaking to a blind man."[74]

THE OPTIC TRACT AND CRANIAL NERVES

Figure 2.5 shows major advances in both illustration technique and anatomy. The upper figure uses transparency to show the relations among the cranial nerves, and the lower figure is an exploded view. Both techniques were used here for the first time. Anatomical drawings did not surpass the clarity of these for centuries.[75, 76]

Galen had described only seven cranial nerves, including the oculomotor but neither the trochlear nor the abducens. As shown in figure 2.5 and rather more clearly in figure 2.6, Leonardo's account of the cranial nerves is an advance over Galen. Here the optic chiasm is illustrated and the olfactory nerves are shown above it. The other nerves appear to be the oculomotor, the abducens, and the ophthalmic branch of the trigeminal,[77, 78] although one observer contends that the latter is the trochlear.[79]

Typically, the cranial nerve sheets contain ambitious programs for future research[80]:

• Draw the nerves which move the eyes in any direction, and its muscles; and do the same with their eyelids, and with the eyebrows, nostrils, cheeks and lips, and everything that moves in a man's face.

• Let the whole ramification of the vessels which serve the brain be made first by itself, separated from the nerves, and then another combined with the nerves.

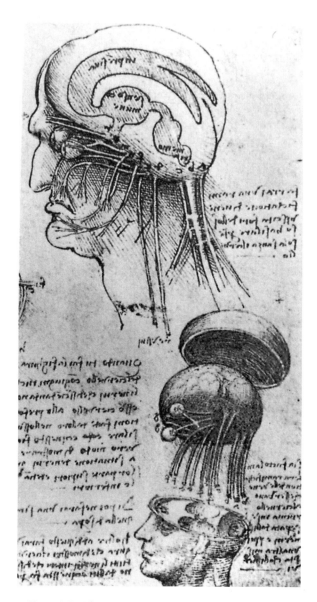

Figure 2.5   The ventricles, optic chiasm, and cranial nerves and (below) exploded view of the skull and brain, ca. 1504–1506. Detail, Schlossmuseum, Weimar.

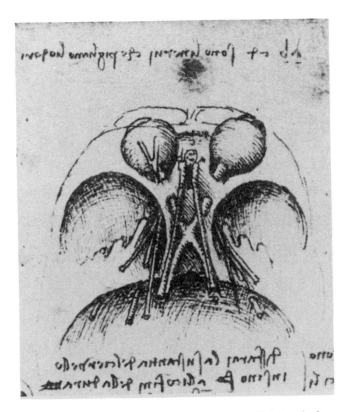

Figure 2.6   The optic and oculomotor nerves, ca. 1504–1506. Detail of W190525.

The Vagus and Hand of an Old Man

Figure 2.7 is a drawing of the right vagus in an old man. How this centenarian came to be his most famous anatomical subject is described by Leonardo as follows:

> And this old man, a few hours before his death told me that he had passed one hundred years, and that he found nothing wrong with his body other than weakness. And thus while sitting upon a

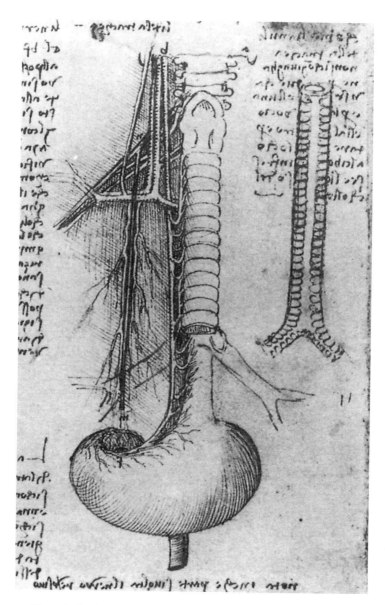

Figure 2.7   The vagus nerve and its recurrent branch innervating the
larynx, trachea, and stomach, ca. 1504–1506. W19050v

bed in the hospital of Santa Maria Nuova in Florence, without any movement or other sign of any mishap he passed out of his life. And I made an anatomy of him in order to see the cause of so sweet a death. This I found to be a fainting away through lack of blood to the artery which nourishes the heart, and other parts below it, which I found very dry, thin and withered. This anatomy I described very diligently and with great ease owing to the absence of fat and humors which greatly hinder the recognition of the parts. (W19027v)

Galen had described in accurate detail the right and left branches of the vagus nerve, known in Leonardo's time as the reversive nerve.[81] Figure 2.7 shows the right branch innervating the larynx, trachea, esophagus, and stomach. Leonardo's interest in the vagus may have been stimulated by Galen's brilliant demonstration that cutting the innervation of the larynx by the recurrent branch of the vagus eliminated vocalization in the pig. (See the bottom panel of figure 1.5.) In the adjacent text Leonardo mentions that the left nerve may innervate the heart. This gives him the occasion to withdraw his earlier Aristotelian belief that the heart is the beginning of life (W19034v):

The heart is not the beginning of life but is a vessel made of dense muscle vivified and nourished by an artery and vein as are the other muscles. It is true that the blood and the artery which purges itself in it are the life and nourishment of the other muscles.

The rest of the text is mostly questions for future research:

Note in what part the left reversive nerve turns and what office it serves. And note the substance of the brain whether it is softer or denser above the origin of the nerve than in other parts. [According to Galen the sensory nerves and the sensory parts of the brain were softer and the motor nerves and the motor parts of the brain were harder. Thus, Leonardo is asking whether the nerve is sensory or motor]. Observe in what way the reversive nerves give sensation to the rings of the trachea and what are the muscles which give movement to the rings to produce a deep, medium or shrill voice. Count the rings of the trachea.

Leonardo is unique up to his time and beyond for constantly counting and measuring in his anatomical studies.

Figure 2.8, also from the centenarian, shows the distribution of the median and ulnar nerves to the palmar aspect of the hand. Unlike the more complicated situation in figure 2.7, this drawing is very accurate.

OPTICS OF THE EYE

Leonardo wrote extensively about light, vision, and the optics of the eye in both an unpublished monograph and in many scattered notes and drawings.[82–86] Although the camera obscura or pinhole camera had been known since late antiquity and was used by Renaissance artists, Leonardo was the first to note its similarity to the eye.[87, 88] He vehemently rejected the implication of this similarity, however; namely, that an inverted image was projected onto the back of the eye and conveyed to the brain. To avoid this unacceptable inversion he tried to develop an optical scheme in which the image was inverted twice in the eye, thereby ending up veridical and ready to be transported to the brain. In fact, he developed about eight such schemes,[89, 90] two of which are shown in figure 2.9. Leonardo actually proposed to build a model to test the lower optical arrangement with his own eye at the site of the optic nerve head of the model.

It is ironic that Leonardo, who presumably easily read his own left–right reversed writing, found it inconceivable that the brain could interpret an inverted image. One hundred years later, Kepler was the first to accept that the image on the black of the eye was indeed inverted since "geometrical laws

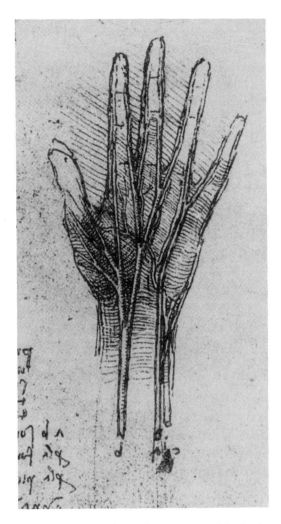

Figure 2.8   The median and ulnar nerves of the hand,
ca. 1504–1509. Detail of W19025v.

Box 2.4 Leonardo on the Difficulties of Anatomy

> "And if you have a love for such [anatomical] things, you will perhaps be hindered by your stomach, and if this does not prevent you, you may perhaps be deterred by the fear of living during the night in the company of quartered and flayed corpses, horrible to see. If this does not deter you, perhaps you lack the good draughtsmanship which appertains to such demonstrations, and if you have the draughtsmanship, it will not be accompanied by a knowledge of perspective. If it were so accompanied, you lack the methods of geometrical demonstration and the method of calculation of the forces and power of the muscles. Perhaps you lack the patience so that you will not be diligent. Whether all these qualities were found in me or not, the hundred and twenty books composed by me will supply the verdict, yes or not. In these pursuits I have been hindered neither by avarice nor by negligence but only by lack of time. Farewell." (W19070v)

leave no choice," and, anyhow, he said, what goes on beyond the retina was not his concern but that of "philosophers."[91]

INFLUENCE OF LEONARDO ON THE COURSE OF NEUROSCIENCE

Leonardo had planned to publish his "120 anatomical notebooks" (see box 2.3) first alone and then as part of a textbook in collaboration with Marc Antonio del Torre, an anatomist and professor of medicine at Padua and later Pavia. However, del Torre died in 1511, before their text was finished (or, as far as we know, started). Leonardo's anatomical drawings had to wait over 200 years for publication. A number of his contemporaries, however, are known to have seen and admired them.[92] Dürer copied several of them, as did several less well-known artists.[93, 94] Leonardo's fame as an artist-anatomist spread throughout northern Italy, and today he is credited with "spearheading the new creative anatomy,"[95] and developing the naturalistic techniques that were made use of by Vesalius (1514–1564) and led to the birth of modern anatomy.[96–99]

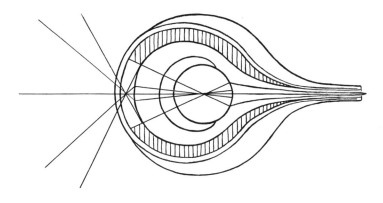

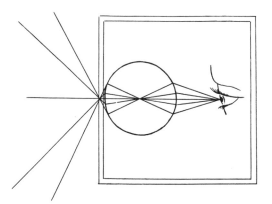

Figure 2.9   Two of Leonardo's attempts to have a double inversion of the image in the eye in order to obtain an upright image at the back of the eye for veridical transmission to the brain. In the lower figure, the eye at the right symbolizes the start of the optic nerve going to the brain (Strong, 1979).

NOTES

1. Clark, 1939.

2. Keele, 1977.

3. Kemp, 1990.

4. McMurrich, 1930.

5. Boring, 1942.

6. Strong, 1979.

7. McMurrich, 1930.

8. Singer, 1957.

9. Herrlinger, 1970.

10. Roberts and Tomlinson, 1992.

11. Herrlinger, 1970. These techniques, however, were common in contemporary treatises on architecture and mechanics that must have been very familiar to Leonardo.

12. O'Malley and Saunders, 1952.

13. Clark, 1935.

14. Reti, 1974.

15. Richter, 1970.

16. MacCurdy, 1954.

17. Singer, 1957.

18. Singer, 1957.

19. Woolam, 1958.

20. Herrlinger, 1970.

21. Roberts and Tomlinson, 1992.

22. Locy, 1911.

23. Singer, 1957.

24. Herrlinger, 1970.

25. Roberts and Tomlinson, 1992.

26. Clayton, 1992.

27. Herrlinger, 1970.

28. Roberts and Tomlinson, 1992.

29. Locy, 1911.

30. Clark, 1939.

31. Singer, 1957.

32. O'Malley and Saunders, 1952.

33. Keele, 1977.

34. McMurrich, 1930.

35. Singer, 1957.

36. O'Malley and Saunders, 1952.

37. Clark, 1935.

38. Reti, 1974.

39. Keele, 1977.

40. O'Malley and Saunders, 1952.

41. Clayton, 1992.

42. O'Malley and Saunders, 1952.

43. Avicenna, 1930; Longrigg, 1993. Curiously, in Taoist sexual theory, semen, conserved by controlling ejaculation, travels in the opposite direction up the spinal cord to the brain (see chapter 1, note 14).

44. Galen, 1956.

45. See chapter 1.

46. MacCurdy, 1954.

47. McMurrich, 1930.

48. MacCurdy, 1954.

49. Richter, 1970.

50. Gross and Bornstein, 1978.

51. Calder, 1970.

52. Mathe, 1980.

53. Keele, 1977.

54. McMurrich, 1930.

55. O'Malley and Saunders, 1952.

56. Clayton, 1992.

57. Boring, 1942.

58. Lindberg, 1976. Le Roy Ladurie's (1997) biography of Platter was recently translated into English.

59. Polyak, 1957.

60. Galen, 1968.

61. Strong, 1979.

62. Lindberg, 1976.

63. Galen, 1956.

64. Galen, 1968.

65. Lindberg, 1976.

66. Polyak, 1957.

67. Gross, 1981.

68. Kemp, 1977.

69. O'Malley and Saunders, 1952.

70. O'Malley and Saunders, 1952.

71. Clayton, 1992.

72. Clark, 1939.

73. Vasari, 1987.

74. McMurrich, 1930.

75. Herrlinger, 1970.

76. Roberts and Tomlinson, 1992.

77. O'Malley and Saunders, 1952.

78. Keele, 1977.

79. Todd, 1991.

80. Lindberg, 1970.

81. Galen, 1956.

82. Strong, 1979.

83. Lindberg, 1976.

84. Ackerman, 1978.

85. Kemp, 1977.

86. Eastwood, 1985.

87. Lindberg, 1976.

88. Lindberg, 1970.

89. Strong, 1979.

90. Eastwood, 1985.

91. Lindberg, 1976.

92. Vasari, 1987.

93. Herrlinger, 1970.

94. Kemp, 1977.

95. Keele, 1964.

96. McMurrich, 1930.

97. Singer, 1957.

98. Keele, 1964.

99. Panofsky, 1962.

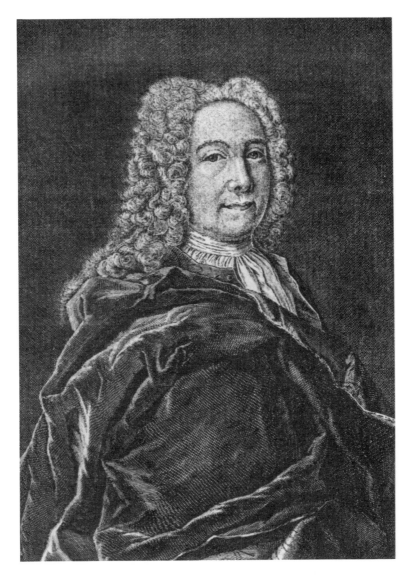

Figure 3.1   Emanuel Swedenborg at age forty-five. From a copper engraving in volume 1 of his *Opera Philosophica et Mineralia* (1734).

Emanuel Swedenborg: A Neuroscientist Before His Time

In 1743, the Swedish nobleman, polymath, and mystic Emanuel Swedenborg began to see and converse with God and angels, and continued to do so until he died thirty years later (figure 3.1). Soon after his death, his followers founded the Swedenborgian Church of the New Jerusalem that continues today as an active Protestant sect. Before his visions began, Swedenborg's interest in the soul led him to study its housing in the brain, and he wrote a set of extraordinary treatises on brain function. These works contained a number of ideas that anticipated modern discoveries by over 100 years. For example, he posited a crucial role of the cerebral cortex in sensory, motor, and cognitive functions, and this during a period in which the cortex was denied any significant functions at all. He even had something very akin to a neuron doctrine, although actual neurons had not been described. Yet, his writings on the brain had no impact on the development of neuroscience.

This chapter begins by reviewing the knowledge of the brain in Swedenborg's time. I then consider his life, his insights into brain function, and the sources of these ideas. I conclude with his influence on the arts and sciences.

NEUROSCIENCE IN THE SEVENTEENTH AND EIGHTEENTH CENTURIES

From the revival of anatomical investigation by Andreas Vesalius of Padua in the sixteenth century until the middle of the nineteenth century, the cerebral cortex was usually considered of little interest. This is indicated by its very name, cortex, Latin for "rind." Vesalius himself thought the function of the cortical convolutions was to allow the blood vessels to bring nutriment to the deeper parts of the brain[1]:

> . . . nature impressed those sinuous foldings throughout the substance of the brain, so that the thin membrane, folded with numerous vessels, could insert itself into the substance of the brain and so to make the cerebral vessels safe by guiding them and so very dexterously administer nourishment.

The first person to examine the cortex microscopically was Marcello Malpighi (1628–1694), professor in Bologna. He saw it as made up of little glands or globules with attached fibers (see figure 1.11)[2]:

> I have discovered in the brain of higher sanguinous animals that the cortex is formed from a mass of very minute glands. These are found in the cerebral gyri which are like tiny intestines and in which the white roots of the nerves terminate or, if you prefer, from which they originate . . . [the globules] are of an oval figure . . . [their] inner portion puts forth a white nervous fibre . . . the white medullary substance of the brain being in fact produced by the connection and fasciculation of many of these.

Similar globules or glandules were also reported by Leewenhoek and other subsequent microscopists.[3] Some historians once thought these pioneers were actually observing cortical pyramidal cells.[4] At least in the case of Malpighi, however, artifacts are now considered a more likely possibility, since Malpighi reported that the globules were more prominent in boiled than fresh tissue. Furthermore, artifacts that look just like Malpighi's globules have been produced by using the methods and instruments he described in detail.[5, 6]

Malpighi's view of the brain as a glandular organ was a common one in the seventeenth and eighteenth centuries. Perhaps a reason for its popularity was that it was consistent with the still persisting views of Aristotle that the brain was a cooling organ, and of the Hippocratic doctors that it was the source of phlegm.[7, 8] The only major figure to attribute any importance to the cerebral cortex was Thomas Willis (1621–1675), professor of natural philosophy at Oxford and author of the first monograph on brain anatomy and physiology[9] (see figure 1.12). Although Willis denied both sensory and motor function to the cerebral cortex, he did attribute to it such higher functions as imagination and memory. However, even this interest in the cerebral cortex dissipated by the end of the seventeenth century.

In the middle of the eighteenth century, physiology was dominated by Albrecht von Haller, professor at Tubingen and later Bern, who was also famous as a botanist, poet, novelist, and politician. Using animals, he tested the "sensibility" of various brain structures with mechanical stimuli such as picking with a scalpel, puncturing with a needle, and pinching with forceps, as well as with chemical stimuli such as silver nitrate, sulfuric acid, and alcohol. With these methods he found the cortex completely insensitive. In contrast, he reported the white matter and subcortical structures such as the thalamus and medulla to be highly sensitive; their stimulation, he said, produced expressions of pain, attempts of the animal to escape, or convulsions.[10]

Haller's ideas on the insensitivity of cortex and the sensitivity of other brain structures were repeatedly confirmed by the experiments of his students, such as J. G. Zinn of "zonule of Zinn" fame, professor of medicine at Gottingen. Describing one such study, Zinn wrote[11]:

> Having cut out a small circular piece of the cranium of a dog with a trephine . . . I pierced the exposed dura mater, touched it with a blade of a scalpel, and poured a solution of mercury sublimate on

it; the animal, however, gave no signs of pain and suffered no convulsions. Since I thought the dog ought to have become apoplectic, I irritated the reflected skin and he showed that he felt pain by giving out a loud cry. . . . Having incised the dura mater, I cut the cortex into pieces, pierced it, irritated it, but the animal showed no sign of pain.

In contrast, when he thrust an instrument through the skull, corpus callosum, and corpus striatum to the base of the brain, as confirmed at autopsy, the dog "howled pitifully . . . vomited repeatedly . . . and died the next day." From observations such as these Haller and his followers concluded that all parts of the cortex were equivalent and were involved in neither sensation nor movement.

In summary, during Swedenborg's time, the cerebral cortex was considered an insensitive rind with no sensory, motor, or higher functions.

SWEDENBORG'S LIFE

Emanuel Swedenborg was born in Stockholm in 1688 of a wealthy mining family that provided him with a lifelong private income. His father was professor of theology at Uppsala, a famous hymn writer, and later a bishop. Swedenborg studied philosophy at Uppsala, but became increasingly involved in science and technology. Among his unrealized schemes were ones for airplanes, submarines, and machine guns. (Do all visionaries dream of flying through the sky, swimming beneath the sea, and efficiently wiping out their enemies, or do Leonardo and Swedenborg have something special in common?) He served on the Board of Mines and made a number of substantial contributions to astronomy, geology, metallurgy, paleontology, and physics.[12–17]

In the 1740s, inspired by studying Newton, Swedenborg began seeking mathematical and mechanical explanations of the origin and nature of the physical and biological universes. He developed a theory of the origin of planets similar to the later and apparently independent ones of Kant and Laplace. He then turned to the problem of the nature of the soul and its relation to the body. This led him to seek the site of the soul in the body and thus to the study of the brain itself[18]:

> I have pursued this [brain] anatomy solely for the purpose of discovering the soul. If I shall have furnished anything of use to the anatomic or medical world it will be gratifying, but still more so if I shall have thrown any light upon the discovery of the soul.

He read widely about the brain in the biological and medical literature of the day, and traveled for extended periods to various countries of western Europe.

His first published writing on the brain was in his *Oeconomia Regni Animalis* of 1740, which was later translated into English as *The Economy of the Animal Kingdom*.[19] By "regni animali" he meant kingdom of the anima or soul; he considered this kingdom or realm to be the human body and, particularly, the brain. By "oeconomia" he meant organization. Thus a better translation of his title might be *Organization of the Body* or, less literally, *The Biological Bases of the Soul*. He also dealt with the brain and sense organs in his second major biological work, *Regnum Animale,*[20] published a few years later. Again, "animale" here means pertaining to the soul.

In 1743 Swedenborg's religious visions began and for the rest of his life he concentrated his energies on religion and spiritual matters. The resulting huge corpus of theological and psychic writings later formed the basis of the Swedenborgian Church. He never returned to his interest in the brain, and much of his writing on the topic remained unpublished in his lifetime. Various religious disputes led him to exile in London, where he died at the age of 83.[21-24]

In the nineteenth century a number of Swedenborg's manuscripts on the brain and sense organs were found by R. L. Tafel in the library of the Swedish Academy of Sciences[25] and published, sometimes first in Latin and then in English. The most important of these, *The Brain,* appeared in 1882 and 1887.[26]

Further translations of Swedenborg's unpublished writings on the brain appeared in the twentieth century, but they were mostly earlier drafts of material already published.[27–29]

VIEWS ON THE CEREBRAL CORTEX

At the very beginning of his biological works Swedenborg announces that his writings will be based primarily on the work of others[30]:

> Here and there I have taken the liberty to throw in the results of
> my experience, but only sparingly . . . I deemed it best to make
> use of the facts supplied by others . . . I laid aside my instruments,
> and restraining my desire for making observations, determined to
> rely rather on the researches of others than to trust my own.

In fact, he very rarely does "throw in" the results of his own work. He provides only a single figure of one of his own brain dissections, that of a drake,[31] and almost no accounts of any of his own experiments or observations.

He begins each section of his biological works with an extensive set of quotations from previous writings on the subject. (These are a marvelous boon for those of us who cannot read medical Latin.) In the next section, entitled "Analysis" or "Induction," he proceeds to weave his own theory of biological structure and function. Such a section from *The Economy of the Animal Kingdom* on "The Cortical Substance of the Brain" characteristically begins, "From the forgoing experience we infer, that the cortex is the principal substance of the brain." In fact, his inference was actually a radical and total departure from the contemporary literature he had just reviewed. Swedenborg then proposed that the cerebral cortex was the most important substance in the brain for sensation, movement, and cognition[32]:

> From the anatomy of the brain it follows that the brain is a
> sensorium commune with respect to its cortical substance . . . since
> to it are referred the impressions of the external sense organs as if

to their one and only internal centre. . . . The cortical substance is also the motorium commune voluntarium for whatever actions are mediated by the nerves and muscles are determined beforehand by the will, that is, by the cortex.

This must be taken as a general principle, that the cortical substance . . . imparts life, that is sensation, perception, understanding and will; and it imparts motion, that is the power of acting in agreement with will and with nature . . .

Central to his brain theory were the cortical globules or glandules described by Malpighi and his successors (see chapter 1 and figure 1.11). In an extraordinary anticipation of the neuron doctrine, Swedenborg suggested that these globules or, as he sometimes called them "cerebellula" (little brains), were functionally independent units that were connected to each other by way of threadlike fibers. These fibers also ran through the white matter and medulla down to the spinal cord, and then by way of the peripheral nerves to various parts of the body. The operations of these cerebellula, he maintained, were the basis of sensation, mentation, and movement.[33]

From each cortical gland proceeds a single . . . nerve fiber; this is carried down into the body, in order that it may take hold of some part of a sensation, or produce some action . . .

SENSORY AND MOTOR FUNCTIONS OF THE CORTEX

Whereas Descartes projected sensory messages to the walls of the ventricle and Willis brought them to the thalamus, Swedenborg thought they terminated in the cerebral cortex, "the seat wherein sensation finally ceases," specifically in the cortical cerebellula[34]:

The external sensations do not travel to any point beyond the cortical cerebellula. This is clear since these are the origin of the nerve fibers.

———

In addition,[35]

> The organ of sight is the eye, while the organ of internal sight is the cortical gland.

He even outlined the pathway from each sense organ to the cortex, a totally unprecedented view and one that was not to reappear until well into the nineteenth century[36]:

> . . . the visual rays flow, by means of the optic nerve, into the thalami nervorum opticorum, and are thence diffused in all directions over the cortex. . . . Also the subtle touches of the olfactory membrane lining the labyrinthine cavities of the nares and the consequent subtle transformation or modifications . . . do not terminate until they arrive . . . in the cortical circumstance. Again the modulations of air, striking upon the delicate . . . internal ear allow themselves to be carried to the medulla and thence toward the supreme cortex. . . . Further, that the tremors excited by the touch of angular bodies in the papillary flesh of the tongue, spread themselves with the sense of taste in a similar manner by their nerves, toward . . . the cortical substance. And that every ruder touch whatever springs up from the surface of the whole, through the medium of the nerves into the medulla spinalis or medulla oblongata, and so into the highly active cineritious [grey] substance and the circumambient cortex of the brain.

He seemed unclear about whether there were discrete cortical areas for every sense or whether all the senses went to the same cortical region, as shown in the following contradictory passages from the same work:

> It is clear from examining the brain that the cortical substances are so wisely arranged as to correspond exactly to every external sen-

sation . . . the general sensorium is designed to receive every species of external sensation—sight, hearing, taste and smell distinctly.

It is the cortical substance collectively that constitutes the internal organism, corresponding to the external organism of the five senses . . . no individual part of the cerebrum corresponds to any sensorial organ of the body; but the cortical substance in general corresponds . . .

The cortex for Swedenborg had motor as well as sensory function, or, in his typically picturesque language[37]:

The cortical glandule is the last boundary where sensations terminate and the last prison house whence the actions break forth; for the fibres, both sensory and motory, begin and end in these glandules.

Remarkably, he had the idea of the somatotopic organization of motor function in the cerebral cortex. He correctly localized control of the foot in the dorsal cortex (he called it the "highest lobe"), the trunk in an intermediate site, and the face and head in the ventral cortex (his third lobe):

. . . the muscle and actions which are in the ultimates of the body or in the soles of the feet depend more immediately upon the highest parts; upon the middle lobe the muscles which belong to the abdomen and thorax, and upon the third lobe those which belong to the face and head; for they seem to correspond to one another in an inverse ratio.

No other suggestion of the somatotopic organization of motor cortex appears until the experiments of Fritsch and Hitzig in 1870.

FURTHER INSIGHTS INTO THE NERVOUS SYSTEM

Swedenborg localized functions in addition to sensation and movement in the cortex. For example, he claimed that the anterior cortex is more important for higher functions than the posterior[38]:

> If this [anterior] portion of the cerebrum . . . is wounded then the internal senses—imagination, memory, thought—suffer; the very will is blunted. . . . This is not the case if the injury is in the back part of the cerebrum.

Frontal lesions are still considered to "blunt the will."

Beyond the cortex, there are a number of other unusual insights about nervous function in Swedenborg's writing. He called the pituitary the "arch gland . . . which receives the whole spirit of the brain and communicates it to the blood." It was the "complement and crown of the whole chymical laboratory of the brain"; and the brain "stimulates the pituitary gland to pour out new life into the blood."[39] Similar views of the pituitary do not appear until the twentieth century.

Swedenborg's view of the circulation of the cerebrospinal fluid was not surpassed until the work of Magendie a 100 years later.[40] He was the first to implicate the colliculi in vision,[41] and in fact the only one until Flourens in the nineteenth century. He suggested that a function of the corpus callosum was for "the hemispheres to intercommunicate with each other."[42] He proposed that a function of the corpus striatum was to take over motor control from the cortex when a movement became a familiar habit or "second Nature."[43]

SOURCES OF SWEDENBORG'S IDEAS ON THE BRAIN

Where did Swedenborg's amazingly prescient views come from? Because of his detailed knowledge of contemporary brain anatomy and physiology, some historians thought that he must have visited brain research laboratories and there carried out dissections or participated in experiments.[44–46] For example, he was in Paris when Pourfour du Petit was conducting experiments on the effects of lesions of the cortex on movement in dogs. Thus, it was proposed that he participated in du Petit's experiments and might have observed the somatotopic organization of motor cortex. Du Petit did realize that the cortex had motor functions, although his claims to this effect were ignored.[47] However, there is no sign that du Petit himself had any notion of the topographic arrangement of motor cortex. Furthermore, Swedenborg's detailed travel diaries provide no evidence that he visited du Petit's or any other laboratory studying the brain during his travels abroad.[48] Visiting churches was more his wont.

The available evidence indicates that Swedenborg's ideas came primarily, if not entirely, from a careful reading and integration of the anatomical, physiological, and clinicopathological literature that was available and that he so copiously quoted.[49, 50] He paid particularly close attention to detailed descriptions and observations rather than simply to the authors' own interpretations and conclusions. Furthermore, he was unusual in attempting to integrate observations of the effects of human brain injury with the details of comparative neuroanatomy.

INFLUENCE AND LACK THEREOF

Swedenborg's writings on religion and spiritualism had an enormous impact on European and American writers and artists. Blake, Yeats, Balzac, the Brownings, Beaudelaire, and Strindberg, for example, all claimed to be particularly influenced by him.[51, 52] In nineteenth-century America his influence was strong among those interested in spiritualism and in transcendentalism.[53] Ralph Waldo Emerson, who was involved in both, declared in 1854, "This age is Swedenborg's."

In spite of his fame in literary, artistic, and religious circles, or perhaps partly because of it, Swedenborg's ideas on the brain remained largely unknown until the twentieth century. The Latin originals of the *Animal Economy* books of the 1740s were not even mentioned in the major physiology textbooks of the following decades, such as those by Haller (1754), Unzer (1771), Prochaska (1784), Blumenbach (1815), Magendie (1826), Bell (1829), or Müller (1840) English translations of Swedenborg that appeared in the 1840s do not seem to have fared any better. They were ignored in the standard physiology textbooks of the day such as Carpenter's (1845) and Todd's (1845), and in Ferrier's (1876) monograph on the brain. Even one of the translators of *The Animal Kingdom,* J. J. G. Wilkinson, a London surgeon, hardly mentioned the brain in either his biography of Swedenborg or his commentary on *The Animal Kingdom.*[54]

Early nineteenth-century reviews of Swedenborg's biological works were few and puzzled. An *Athenaeum* reviewer in 1844 noted that *The Animal Kingdom* "will startle the physiologist and [contains] many assumptions he will be far from conceding."[55] The most positive responses seem to have come from books on phrenology[56] or mesmerism.[57]

However, by the time the first volume of *The Brain* was published in 1882, the Zeitgeist had radically changed. Fritsch and Hitzig (1870) had discovered motor cortex, and the race to establish the location of the visual and other sensory cortices was well under way. Now Swedenborg's ideas on the brain made sense, and both volumes received long rave reviews in *Brain,*[58] where the reviewer called it "one of the most remarkable books we have seen" and noted that:

> . . . it appears to have anticipated some of the most modern discoveries [on the brain] but that because of its metaphysical, ontological, theological phraseology . . . if it had not been that attention was arrested and enchanted by finding so many anticipations of scientific discoveries by as much as 120 or 130 years, we should have been tempted to throw aside the book as beyond our province, if not hopelessly unintelligible.

Nevertheless, Swedenborg's writings on the brain seem to have disappeared from sight again, not being mentioned in Foster's (1893) or Schäfer's (1900) authoritative textbooks of physiology, in Ferrier's (1886) or Campbell's (1905) monographs on the brain, in the history of the field by Foster,[59] or even the massive two-volume one by Soury.[60]

In 1901 Swedenborg's extraordinary anticipations on the brain were finally publicized by the great historian of neuroscience Max Neuberger, professor of the history of medicine in Vienna.[61] As a result, they became the subject of further accounts by neuroanatomists and historians, particularly Swedish ones.[62–66] In 1910 a conference of 400 delegates from 14 countries was held in London in honor of his many contributions to science, philosophy and theology.[67]

WHY WAS SWEDENBORG SO IGNORED?

Several examples of biologists were so ahead of their time that their writings were read but not understood by their contemporaries. Appreciation of their ideas had to wait until further advances closed the gap between them and lesser mortals. Arguably, the most famous example was Gregor Mendel.[68] Sometimes it is an otherwise well-known and successful scientist who has certain ideas that are only grasped in later generations. Outstanding examples of this are Darwin's concept of the irregularly branching and nonhierarchical process of natural selection[69] and Claude Bernard's maxim on the necessity of a constant internal milieu for the development of a complex nervous system.[70]

Swedenborg's case is more extreme. There is little evidence that contemporary physiologists and anatomists even read his writings on the brain. He never held an academic post or had students, colleagues, or scientific correspondents. He never carried out any systematic empirical work on the brain, and his speculations were in the form of baroque and grandiose pronouncements embedded in lengthy books on the human soul by one whose fame was soon to be that of a mystic or madman. Even he seems to have lost interest in his ideas on the brain, as he never finished or published many of his manuscripts on the subject. Furthermore, some of his more advanced theories, such as on the organization of motor cortex or the functions of the pituitary gland, did not appear in print until after they were no longer new. As a neuroscientist, Swedenborg failed to publish, and as a neuroscientist he certainly perished.

NOTES

1. Vesalius, 1966.

2. Malpighi, 1666.

3. Meyer, 1971.

4. Nordenskiold, 1928.

5. Meyer, 1971.

6. Clarke and Bearn, 1968.

7. Gross, 1995.

8. Gross, 1987b.

9. Willis, 1664.

10. Neuburger, 1981.

11. Neuburger, 1981.

12. Jonsson, 1971.

13. Dingle, 1958.

14. Toksvig, 1848.

15. Transactions of the International Swedenborg Congress, 1911.

16. Wilkinson, 1849.

17. Tafel, 1877.

18. Swedenborg, 1887.

19. Swedenborg, 1845–1846.

20. Swedenborg, 1843–1844.

21. Jonsson, 1971.

22. Toksvig, 1848.

23. Wilkinson, 1849.

24. Tafel, 1877.

25. Tafel, 1877.

26. Swedenborg, 1882–1887.

27. Swedenborg, 1938.

28. Swedenborg, 1922.

29. Swedenborg, 1914.

30. Swedenborg, 1845–1846.

31. Swedenborg, 1845–1846.

32. Swedenborg, 1845–1846.

33. Swedenborg, 1922.

34. Swedenborg, 1845–1846.

35. Swedenborg, 1882–1887.

36. Swedenborg, 1845–1846.

37. Swedenborg, 1882–1887.

38. Swedenborg, 1882–1887.

39. Swedenborg, 1882–1887.

40. Squires, 1940.

41. Swedenborg, 1882–1887.

42. Swedenborg, 1882–1887.

43. Akert and Hammond, 1962.

44. Akert and Hammond, 1962.

45. Retzius, 1908.

46. Acton, 1938.

47. Neuburger, 1981.

48. Tafel, 1877.

49. Ramstrom, 1910.

50. Ramstrom, 1911.

51. Jonsson, 1971.

52. Toksvig, 1848.

53. Novak, 1969.

54. Wilkinson, 1846.

55. Anonymous, 1844.

56. Combe, 1852.

57. Bush, 1847.

58. Rabagliati, 1984, 1988.

59. Foster, 1901.

60. Soury, 1899.

61. Neuburger, 1901.

62. Nordenskiold, 1928.

63. Transactions . . . , 1911.

64. Retzius, 1908.

65. Ramstrom, 1910.

66. Norrving and Sourander, 1989.

67. Transactions . . . , 1911.

68. See chapter 1, note 113.

69. Mayr, 1982.

70. Olmstead, 1967.

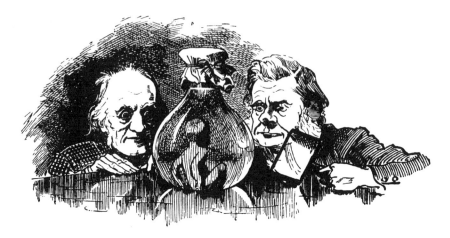

Figure 4.1   Richard Owen (left) and Thomas Huxley examining a water baby. Drawing by Linley Sambourne from a 1916 edition of Charles Kingley's novel for children, *Water Babies,* originally published in 1863. It includes a spoof of the hippocampus minor controversy.

The Hippocampus Minor and Man's Place in Nature: A Case Study in the Social Construction of Neuroanatomy

In midnineteenth-century Britain, the possibility of evolution and particularly the evolution of humans from apes was vigorously contested. Among the leading antievolutionists was the celebrated anatomist and paleontologist Richard Owen, and among the leading defenders of evolution was T. H. Huxley (figure 4.1). The central dispute between them on human evolution was whether or not man's brain was fundamentally unique.

This chapter considers the background of this controversy, the origin and fate of the term hippocampus minor, why this structure became central to the question of human evolution, and how Huxley used it to support both Darwinism and the political ascendancy of Darwinians. The account illustrates both the extraordinary persistence of ideas in biology and the role of the political and social matrix in the study of the brain.

Evolution and Victorian Politics

For several decades before the publication of the *Origin of Species* in 1859, debate raged in Britain over the possibility of the transmutation of species and, especially, of an ape origin for humans. At the beginning of the century J.B. Lamarck elaborated the first coherent theory of evolution and unambiguously included humans. He thought that evolution involved continuous upward progress, an inevitable transformation of lower into upper forms of life. His "progressivism," as well as his materialism and his belief in the inheritance of acquired characteristics, made Lamarck very appealing to the London and Edinburgh radicals of the day. They took his idea that biological evolution implies progress and improvement and applied it to society to demand social evolution and social progress. Some of the transformations they advocated were the end of aristocratic and established church privilege, introduction of universal suffrage, reform of medical care and medical education (many were physicians), education for women, and similar radical reformist notions. Correspondingly, the conservative Oxbridge scientist-clergymen who dominated early Victorian science saw Lamarck as a direct threat to the established order of Church and State.[1]

Evolutionary ideas and their radical political and theological implications became more widespread with the publication in 1844 of *Vestiges of the Natural History of Creation* by Robert Chambers, a scientific amateur who published anonymously because of the very real threats of blasphemy laws and economic and political persecution.[2] *Vestiges* argued for both cosmic and biological evolution, and adopted Lamarck's idea that evolution implied improvement. Chambers's arguments for biological evolution included the location of simpler fossils in older strata, the fundamentally similar anatomical organization of all groups of animals, and tendencies of embryos to go through stages similar to their putative ancestors. The book was a sensational best-seller, with some 24,000 copies sold in the next ten years compared with 9,500 for Darwin's *Origin* over a similar period. That Chambers was a successful publisher, expert in marketing popular science, undoubtedly helped.[3]

The scientific establishment reacted rather violently to *Vestiges*. Adam Sedgwick, professor of geology at Cambridge, president of the Geological Society, and a future president of the British Association for the Advancement of Science, wrote a 500-page plus review of this "beastly book" to place "an iron heel upon the head of the filthy abortion and put an end to its crawlings" in which he made clear that the problem was not merely scientific:

———

> The world cannot bear to be turned upside down . . . I can see
> nothing but ruin and confusion in such a creed. . . . If current in
> society it will undermine the whole moral and social fabric and
> inevitably will bring discord and deal mischief in its train . . .

In a letter to Charles Lyell he went further:

> if the book be true . . . religion is a lie; human law is a mass of
> folly, and a base injustice; morality is moonshine; our labours for
> the black people of Africa were the works of madmen . . .

The Rev. Sedgwick seems to have been particularly incensed that a book for
the general public (and therefore for women too) dealt with such topics as
pregnancy and abortion, and he cautioned that[4]:

> our glorious maidens and matrons . . . not soil their fingers with
> the dirty knife of an anatomist neither may they poison the strings
> of joyous thought and modest feeling by listening to the seductions
> of this author . . .

T. H. Huxley, later to be the great battler for evolution, was almost as brutal,
his review using such terms as "foolish fantasies," "pretentious nonsense," and
"work of fiction."[5]

Despite the establishment attacks on it, *Vestiges* was a popular success, so
much so that Disraeli parodied its fashion in middle-class salons in his 1847
novel *Tancred*.[6] Chambers gave ammunition to the radicals and socialists, who
used the book's ideas of biological progress to demand social progress.[7] Chambers certainly made many factual errors and uncritical speculations, yet, as Mayr
wrote, "it was he who saw the forest where all the great British scientists of
his period (except Darwin) only saw the trees." Chambers's book helped make
both the scientific and lay world ready for the far more coherent and compelling
arguments in the *Origin,* a debt that Darwin later acknowledged. Furthermore,

———

it influenced A.R. Wallace, codiscoverer of natural selection. It may also have had a significant effect on Darwin himself, as Darwin's son Francis later reported that his father's copy was well read and annotated.[8]

Lamarck's and Chambers's explicit and graphic descriptions of the transformation of ape into human piqued popular interest in the apes and monkeys Victorian imperialism was now bringing to Britain in increasing numbers. Chimpanzees were dressed in human clothes at the London Zoo, and anthropomorphic prints of them implied the proximity that these authors made explicit.[9] This "beastialization" of man implicitly supported the idea of evolution, which in turn implied materialism and social transformation, thereby threatening the established church and state. The leading figure to combat this threat was Professor (later Sir) Richard Owen, and he was superbly placed to do so.

OWEN SEPARATES MAN FROM THE APES

Owen had been elected to the Royal Society by the age of thirty, was Hunterian Professor at the Royal College of Surgeons, and became superintendent of the Natural History Department of the British Museum, which gave him a monopoly on dissecting animals that died in the London Zoo. He was easily England's leading paleontologist and anatomist, the "British Cuvier." He also became socially well connected; he received a London residence from the queen, dined with Prince Albert and the Prince of Wales, and lectured to the Royal Children on zoology. Nor was his political conservatism only theoretical: when the Chartists (advocating universal male suffrage, equal electoral districts, the end of property qualifications for members of parliament, and similar reforms) were thought to threaten London with their militant marches and violent demonstrations, he joined the militia of urban gentry to defend, quite literally, the status quo.[10]

In the years before the publication of the *Origin,* Owen wrote a series of papers comparing the muscles and bones of apes with those of humans. He stressed the differences between them and used these differences to argue for

---

their independent origin and the impossibility of the transmutation of one into the other. One major line of argument was that the anatomical details of the leg and foot of the orang-utan were quite incompatible with the animal standing erect and walking like a human. Lamarck's simple-minded notion of an ape climbing down from a tree and becoming a man was clearly wrong. Another theme concerned the similarities of the heads and faces of humans and chimpanzees. Prior to Owen's work, infant but not mature chimpanzees had been described; infant chimps have faces and heads very similar to those of human children (a phenomenon now known as neoteny), making a close relationship plausible. Owen obtained the skull of a mature chimp and, describing its bony ridges for holding strong jaw muscles, its protruding jaws, and its threatening canines, contended that it was far more bestial than a baby chimp's and too much so to be a close relative of man.[11]

Then, at the peak of his career, he wrote a paper that within a few years was repudiated by the scientific community and ridiculed in the popular press, and fixed him in the history books for an egregious triplet of errors rather than for his over 600 scientific papers, many of which had made significant contributions. The paper, "On the Characters, Principles of Division and Primary Groups of the Class Mammalia," was read at a meeting of the Linnean Society and again as the Rede lecture at Cambridge University, on the occasion of Owen receiving the first honorary degree ever given by that university.[12] The startling part of this paper was a new classification of mammals that stressed the gap between human and ape. Its timing was probably spurred by Owen's realization that Darwin was about to publish his book on transmutation.

In the eighteenth century, Linnaeus had put men, apes, monkeys, and lemurs (and bats) into a single order, Primates, and this grouping, minus bats, had been accepted by most zoologists. Owen now rejected this dominant tradition and placed humans apart from all other primates and indeed from all other mammals in a separate subclass, the Archencephala ("ruling brain"). He did so on three anatomical criteria, all of them concerning the brain. Presumably, he chose brain structures because of the human's mental uniqueness and superiority. Furthermore, to strengthen his theory of the lack of continuity between man and animals, he maintained that these three structures were actually found exclusively in humans, rather than merely being larger or different than in animals. He sought a truly qualitative difference between man and beast and he wanted it based on anatomical science.

The first fundamental difference he claimed was that only in the human does the "posterior lobe" (i.e., the posterior of the cerebrum) extend beyond the cerebellum. He supported this with illustrations contrasting the brain of a chimpanzee with that of a Negro. The comparison of a Negro brain with an ape brain was common in the nineteenth and extended well into the twentieth century. The rationale was that as the "lowest" race with "therefore" the least developed brains, blacks were the most appropriate comparison with animals. This view was nearly universal among nineteenth-century scientists, even those such as Darwin who were ardent abolitionists.[13] The most often illustrated nonwhite brain was that of the famous "Hottentot Venus" (Saartjie Baartman), who was exhibited in London and Paris and described in detail by many of the leading anatomists of the day, including Paul Broca and Georges Cuvier, both when she was alive and after her death and dissection.[14]

The second difference proposed by Owen was that only humans have a posterior horn or cornu in their lateral ventricles. The third and most important difference was that only humans have a hippocampus minor. These extraordinary claims were supported by no citations to the literature, no brain sections, and no illustrations other than those just mentioned. Near the end of the paper, just in case the reader overlooked the importance of the missing hippocampus minor and the other supposed deprivations of the animal brain, Owen wrote: "Thus, [man] fulfills his destiny as the supreme master of this earth and of the lower creation." When Darwin read Owen's paper he commented, "I cannot swallow Man . . . [so] . . . distinct from a Chimpanzee . . . I wonder what a Chimpanzee wd say to this?"[15]

In the following section I describe what the hippocampus minor actually is, since the term has disappeared from contemporary neuroanatomy. Next I discuss Huxley's challenge to Owen's new classification of man and how he used the hippocampus minor to repudiate Owen and irreparably damage his scientific credibility, thereby facilitating the acceptance of Darwin's ideas. After I consider the origins of Owen's criteria for humanness, I address some consequences and implications of the debate.

The Hippocampus Minor

The hippocampus minor is a ridge in the floor of the posterior horn of the lateral ventricle caused by the deep inward penetration of the calcarine fissure. The original term for the hippocampus minor was calcar avis, and this is the one that is used today. It is not easily visible in coronal, sagittal, or horizontal sections but is clearly discernable on blunt dissection, exposing the posterior horn from above (figure 4.2). Where did this physically unimpressive and, to the contemporary neuroscientist, unimportant, structure get its names?

In a top-down dissection through the human brain, the hippocampus is a particularly prominent feature on the floor of the lateral ventricle. It received its modern name from Aranzi (Arantius), a student of Vesalius in 1564, because its features reminded him of the sea horse, or hippocampus. Another somewhat less prominent structure, also visible in this approach, is a ridge on the floor of the posterior horn of the ventricle. As it resembles the spur on a bird's leg, this ridge was named calcar avis, from the Latin for cock's spur. In systemizing brain nomenclature in 1786, Vicq d'Azyr renamed these two ventricular structures. The calcar avis was named the hippocampus minor, and the hippocampus became the hippocampus major. Things got a bit bizarre for a while when Meyer in 1779 erroneously used the word hippopotamus instead of hippocampus, which was maintained by several authors until Burdach straightened things out in 1829.[16]

The terms calcar avis and hippocampus minor continued to be used interchangeably until the later part of the nineteenth century, when the latter term disappeared, having been officially expunged in the 1895 edition of *Nomina Anatomica*. This disappearance may have been related to the ridicule and controversy that swirled around the term in the debates we are about to relate. At this time hippopotamus again was substituted for hippocampus, but

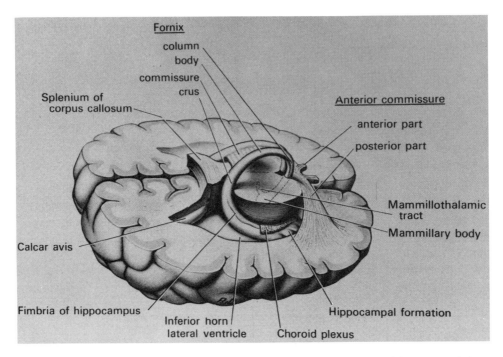

Figure 4.2 Modern drawing of a human brain dissection showing the hippocampal formation and the calcar avis in the floor of the lateral ventricle (from Carpenter and Sutin, 1983, with permission).

in jest, as in Charles Kingsley's *Water Babies,*[17] as we will see. The contrasting designation hippocampus major for what is now called the hippocampus lingered for a few more years, and then also fell out of use. Whereas the hippocampus minor was virtually absent from anatomy textbooks by the turn of the century, it survived in those more conservative sources, dictionaries (e.g., *Webster's New International Dictionary,* 2nd ed., 1957), and encyclopedias (e.g., *Encyclopedia Britannica,* 13th ed., 1926).

Before returning to the fate of Owen's proposals for the hippocampus minor it may be helpful to summarize the state of contemporary knowledge of brain function. The year 1858 can be viewed as a time after the fertilization but before the birth of modern neuroscience. The phrenological movement initiated by Gall and Spurzheim at the turn of the nineteenth century had popularized the idea of the cerebrum as a collection of organs with different psychological functions, and focused attention on the functions of the cerebral cortex. Gall's errors of equating skull features with brain morphology had been realized in the scientific community, and the search for correlations between the site of cerebral damage and symptom had begun in humans and animals. Flourens's experimental work on pigeons and other animals in the 1820s had simultaneously demolished the extreme localization of phrenology and made the idea of more limited localization of function readily acceptable.[18] However, at the time of Owen's paper, no convincing evidence existed for the specific functions of any portion of the mammalian cerebrum; the hippocampus minor was no more a terra incognita than any other area.

In the years immediately after Owen's paper, three crucial events occurred in the understanding of brain function. The first was Broca's demonstration in 1861 of an area critical for speech in the left frontal lobe. It was the first generally accepted localization of psychological function in the human brain and it was viewed at the time as a vindication of Gall. The second was Fritsch and Hitzig's production of specific movements by electrical stimulation of discrete motor centers of the cortex in 1870. The third was the discovery of the sensory areas of the cortex, which followed soon thereafter.[19]

T. H. Huxley as Young Bulldog

Thomas Henry Huxley was twenty-one years Owen's junior and was hostile to the older scientist almost from the beginning of his scientific career. In 1850 Huxley had just returned from a four-year voyage aboard the *H.M.S. Rattlesnake*. Unlike Darwin's status on the *Beagle* as gentleman naturalist, Huxley had been a lowly assistant surgeon, and what research he did was on his own time. It was good enough, particularly that on coelenterates, that he was elected to the Royal Society in 1851. Yet, for several years after returning, he was without a job or research funds (but with a fiancée waiting in Australia).[20]

In this period, Owen supported Huxley's candidacy for the Royal Society and wrote several letters of recommendation for him for various teaching or research posts. At the end of 1852, Huxley wrote Owen for yet another letter of recommendation, this time to the Navy. When Owen failed to answer in the next ten days, Huxley wrote again, and still did not receive an answer. Four days later the men happened to meet and Huxley described the confrontation in a letter in a way that nicely epitomizes the personalities of the junior and senior scientists[21]:

> Of course I was in a considerable rage. . . . I was going to walk past, but he stopped me, and in the blandest and most gracious manner said, "I have received your note. I shall *grant* it." The phrase and the implied condescension were quite "touching," so much that if I stopped for a moment longer I must knock him into the gutter. I therefore bowed and walked off.

Owen sent the recommendation a few days later and the Navy gave Huxley funds to complete publication of his research from the voyage. Yet during this time Huxley repeatedly attacked Owen, but only privately, writing, for example, that "Owen is both feared and hated" and that "he [Huxley] felt it necessary always to be on guard against him [Owen]." He even thought that Owen was blocking publication of his papers and taking his grant money, both charges apparently without justification. He wrote to his sister in 1852[22]:

> Let him [Owen] beware. . . . On my subjects I am his master and am quite ready to fight. . . . And although he has a bitter pen . . . I can match him . . .

Finally, in 1854 Huxley secured a position teaching natural history at the Government School of Mines. He kept it for another thirty years, eventually turning down chairs at Oxford and Harvard, among other places. By this time the school had become the Royal School of Science and would eventually become Imperial College. No longer needing job references from Owen, Huxley's attacks on his senior became more public. Huxley's scientific critiques of Owen in the late 1850s included ones on the subjects of parthenogenesis, on the presence of an anus in a group of brachiopods, on Owen's classification of Invertebrates, and on his comparative anatomy textbook. With Owen in the chair, Huxley's Croonian lecture to the Royal Society in 1859 was a violent critique of Owen's theory that the skull is composed of fused vertebrae. This was part of Owen's theory of archetypes, that there was a basic pattern to which all vertebrates conformed. This theory largely derived from the idealistic morphology of Naturphilosophie, whose origin was the Platonic Romanticism of Goethe and Schiller. Contemporary skull nomenclature stems from this effort of Owen.[23]

The final personal breach between Huxley and Owen came in 1857 when Owen gave a successful series of lectures on paleontology at the Government School of Mines.[24] They were attended by various luminaries such as the Duke of Argyll (then Postmaster General and later president of the Royal Society), Sir Charles Lyell, and David Livingston. In this connection Owen listed himself in a medical directory as "Professor of Comparative Anatomy and Paleontology" in the School of Mines. Huxley was infuriated at this intrusion into his territory and complained to the editor of the directory:

Mr. Owen holds no appointment whatever at the Govt. School of Mines, and as I am the Professor of General Natural History (which includes Comparative Anatomy and Paleontology) in that Institution you will observe that the statement . . . is calculated to do me injury.

To a friend, Huxley wrote[25]:

I have now done with him, personally. I would as soon acknowledge a man who had attempted to obtain my money on false pretenses.

Although scientific controversy tended to be much more openly nasty in Victorian England than it is today, the Owen-Huxley antagonism was extreme even by standards of the time, and it had far from peaked at the time of this territorial dispute. Huxley's youthful arrogance, hot temper, and anticlericism, and Owen's stubbornness, superciliousness, and religiosity served to exaggerate their scientific differences. The fact that both came from lower middle-class backgrounds, and Owen eagerly sought and Huxley tended to resist social ascent, probably further exacerbated their differences. Of course, in a few decades the amateur naturalist-clergyman Oxbridge establishment would give way to the professional scientist establishment with the Right Honorable Huxley and his friends in the X Club at its very center.[26]

By the end of the 1850s, under Darwin's tutorial, Huxley was gradually accepting the idea of transmutation and what it implied about the origin of humankind; his prepublication reading of the *Origin* finally made him a total convert to the idea of evolution. Like most of Darwin's contemporaries, however, he never really accepted and probably never grasped Darwin's core contribution, the concept of natural selection operating on random variation.[27]

THE OXFORD MEETING OF THE BRITISH ASSOCIATION, 1860

The British Association for the Advancement of Science was the largest scientific organization in Britain and its annual meetings were the most public. Its meetings were reported and commented on in the press, even in the popular dailies. The serious weeklies, particularly the *Athenaeum,* usually carried detailed reports of the major papers presented. In anticipation of the 1858 annual meeting in Leeds, Huxley had written "The interesting question arises, shall I have a row with the great O. there?" Two years later he got what was obviously his wish.

The 1860 meeting in Oxford of this "parliament of science" was the first after the publication of the *Origin of Species* and, as a result, interest in it was high among the lay and scientific public. By this time the *Origin* had been discussed in detail in virtually all the serious press. Reviews covered the spectrum from slashing attacks by Owen (thinly anonymously) in the *Edinburgh*

Review and by Samuel Wilberforce, Bishop of Oxford, in the *Quarterly Review* to the undiluted enthusiasm of T. H. Huxley in both the very respectable *Times* (anonymously) and the radical *Westminster Review*. Darwin called Owen's assessments "extremely malignant," Wilberforce's "uncommonly clever," and Huxley's "brilliant." As had become his custom for virtually all public scientific meetings because of his chronic illness, Darwin himself did not attend, but eagerly awaited news particularly from his closest colleagues, botanist J. D. Hooker and Huxley.[28]

On Thursday, June 28, the opening day of the meeting, after a paper entitled, "On the Final Causes of the Sexuality of Plants with Particular Reference to Mr. Darwin's Work," the chair called on Huxley for his comments. According to a report in the *Athenaeum,* the leading contemporary intellectual weekly, Huxley declined to comment because:

> he felt a general audience in which sentiment would unduly interfere with intellect, was not the public before which such a discussion should be carried out.

Owen then asked for the floor to present facts "by which the public could come to some conclusions . . . of the truth of Mr. Darwin's theory." He then repeated his argument that the brain of the gorilla was more different from that of man than from that of the lowest primate particularly because only man had a posterior lobe, a posterior horn, and a hippocampus minor. Hence, the descent of humans from apes, a crucial implication of Darwin's ideas, was impossible.

Then Huxley rose and "denied altogether that the difference between the brain of the gorilla and man was so great," making a "direct and unqualified contradiction" of Owen. In support of his position, Huxley cited previous studies and promised to defend his arguments in detail elsewhere.[29] He did so, as we will see, repeatedly over the next three years.

The next day Huxley was planning to leave the meeting because Bishop Wilberforce was rumored to be planning to "smash Darwin," and Huxley was afraid that the "promised debate would be merely an appeal to prejudice in a mixed audience before which the scientific arguments of the Bishop's opponents would be at the utmost disadvantage." The Bishop had a first-class degree in mathematics, which supposedly made him an authority on science. Owen was staying with Wilberforce, prepping him for the debate, just as he had helped him with a very negative review of the *Origin*. That afternoon Huxley ran into Robert Chambers, who by now was generally believed to be the author of *Vestiges,* the revolutionary tract on evolution. On hearing that Huxley was planning to leave, Chambers "vehemently" urged him not to "desert them." Huxley recalled replying, "Oh! If you are going to take it that way I'll come."[30]

The next day the lecture room was packed, and when Dr. Draper from New York finished his lecture, "The Intellectual Development of Europe Considered with Reference to the Views of Mr. Darwin and Others that the Progression of Organisms Is Determined by Law," the Bishop of Oxford rose and spoke for "full half an hour . . . ridiculing Darwin badly and Huxley savagely," and in general repeating arguments from his review of the *Origin*. Then turning to Huxley, and referring to the clash two days earlier between Owen and Huxley over brain anatomy and the relatedness of man and ape, "he begged to know was it through his grandfather or his grandmother that he claimed descent from a monkey?" Huxley supposedly turned to his neighbor saying, "The Lord has delivered him into mine hands."

Huxley rose, calmly, in his memory, but "white with anger" according to others, and defended Darwin's theory as "the best explanation of the origin of species which had yet been offered." He concluded with the most famous repartee in the history of science, that:

> he was not ashamed to have a monkey for his ancestor; but he would be ashamed to be connected with a man who used great gifts to obscure the truth.

Some accounts were stronger ending:

———

I should feel it a shame to have sprung from one who prostituted the gifts of culture and eloquence to the service of prejudice and of falsehood.

According to one report:

as the point became clear there was a great burst of applause, one lady fainted and had to be carried out, I for one jumped out of my seat, no one who was present can ever forget the impression it made.

Other speakers followed, including FitzRoy, now Admiral, formerly Captain of the *Beagle,* regretting the publication of Darwin's book, and John Lubbock, pioneering ethologist, accepting the Darwinian hypothesis as the best available. Speaking last and at length, J. D. Hooker gave a detailed refutation of Wilberforce and defense of Darwin using his expertise as a botanist and biogeographer.

Years later, particularly after accounts of these events were published by Huxley and Darwin's sons, the exchange between Huxley and Wilberforce took on a exaggerated mythic existence as the "Great Battle in the War between Science and Religion," the most famous nineteenth-century battle after Waterloo, in which Huxley committed "forensic murder" and Wilberforce "involuntary martyrdom." At the time, however, each man believed himself the victor. Furthermore, Hooker thought he, rather than Huxley, had demolished Wilberforce. The audience seems to have been divided among these three views; the *Athenaeum* summarized it all as "uncommonly lively." Jensen critically reviewed the contemporary reports, the recollections of the participants, and the large and ever growing secondary literature on this so-called debate.[31]

THE "BULLDOG" AND "GLADIATOR-GENERAL FOR SCIENCE" ATTACKS[32]

Huxley had been waiting and preparing for his attack on Owen at the British Association meeting for some time. As soon as he read Owen's new classification scheme separating humans from other primates on the basis of brain structure, he began systematically to dissect monkey brains. He soon realized the magnitude of Owen's errors and saw his opportunity to "nail . . . [Owen] . . . that menditous humbug . . . like a kite to the barn door." He said nothing publicly until his contradiction in the opening session of the 1860 Oxford meeting. After that, as promised, he began to attack Owen's claims in print and with a vengeance. He used his new journal, *Natural History Review,* as a major platform. He had just founded it as a pro-Darwin and anticlerical ("episcopo-phagous") organ.[33]

The opening of Huxley's campaign came in 1861 in the first issue.[34] There he attacked the three claims of Owen, that only man's cerebrum covered the cerebellum (the posterior lobe), that only man had a posterior horn in his lateral ventricle, and that only man had a hippocampus minor. He did so with a barrage of citations, quotations, and personal communications from leading anatomists in Britain and abroad. Huxley was interested in doing more than proving Owen wrong. He wanted to prove him dishonest as well. Thus, he put great emphasis on quoting three particular sources that Owen must have known about, and stated that in failing to mention them he was "guilty of willful and deliberate falsehood."

The first of these sources was Owen himself in a monograph that was a major factor in establishing the man's anatomical reputation, and that antedated *Vestiges* and Owen's antipathy to transmutation. In it Owen briefly notes that the cerebral hemispheres of the baboon and chimpanzee extend beyond the cerebellum.[35]

The second authority was F. Tiedemann, a distinguished German anatomist from whose 1836 paper in the *Philosophical Transactions* Owen copied, without attribution, the drawing of the Negro brain in his classification paper. Huxley quoted earlier papers by Tiedemann describing, in infrahuman primates, the cerebrum extending beyond the cerebellum and a posterior horn in the lateral ventricle. He was a little misleading here, since in the paper from which Owen obtained the drawing of the Negro brain, illustrations of orang-utan and chimpanzee brains actually show the cerebrum not extending beyond the cerebellum. Huxley also rather quickly passed over Tiedemann's earlier failure to find a hippocampus minor in any animal other than man.[36] (The point of Tiedemann's 1836 paper, incidentally, was to argue, rather iconoclastically, for the neuroanatomical, intellectual, and moral equality of whites and blacks. To support their anatomical equality, he showed the brain of the "Hottentot Venus" and claimed, unlike several other anatomists, that it is essentially identical to the brains of Europeans. To support his claim of intellectual and moral equality, Teidemann provided a list of distinguished black clergyman, intellectuals, artists, and political leaders.)

The third source Huxley used to impugn Owen's integrity was a paper by Dutch anatomists J. L. C. Schroeder van der Kolk and W. Vrolik.[37] Again Owen must have seen this paper since that is where he obtained, again without attribution, his illustration of a chimpanzee brain showing its cerebellum uncovered by the cerebrum. In this paper the authors clearly described a posterior horn and a hippocampus minor in the chimpanzee. As to their figure showing the exposed cerebellum, Huxley quoted Gratiolet, the leading brain anatomist of the day, that this specific figure was greatly distorted and misleading because of the way the brain was removed from the skull. Tiedemann's drawings of both the orang-utang and the chimpanzee showed the same distortion.[38] This must have been a common error and not quite the absurdity Huxley claimed. Animals, and certainly rare apes, were not perfused with a fixative for anatomical purposes when they were still alive, as is done today, under anesthesia, for optimal histological fixation. Rather, when they died, usually in a zoo, their brains were removed and placed in a preservative. Under these conditions the kind of distortion that misled Owen and his sources must have been common indeed.

Owen's Linnean (1858) and Rede lectures (1859) on the classification of mammals were identical except for a footnote missing from the latter. In that note Owen said he was unable to shut his eyes to the "all-pervading similitude of structure which makes the determination of the differences between" human and chimpanzee "so difficult." He presumably originally included this comment to stress the importance of his three new cerebral criteria for distinguishing human and ape, but then may have omitted it in the republication because he realized it undercut his theory. In any case Huxley, here and many times again, reveled in quoting this footnote, which he treated as the ultimate hoisting petard.

At the end of his *Natural History Review* paper, Huxley readily admitted several differences between the human brain and that of the higher apes, such as size, relative proportions of different parts, and the complexity and number of convolutions. These he believed were "of no very great value" because they were the same as those between the brains of the "highest" and "lowest" human races "though more in degree." He then took exception to Tiedemann's view that the brain of a black was no different from that of a European, since this weakened his view of the continuity between human and ape, with the "lower" races of man intermediate. In any case, he concluded, the brains of monkeys "differ far more widely from the brain of an orang than the brain of an orang differs from that of man" and therefore, Owen's dividing the two by cerebral characters was wrong.

As soon as this paper appeared Huxley sent the "Lord Bishop of Oxford" a reprint of it with a short note to "draw attention" to it as a "full justification for contradicting Owen at the Oxford British Association meeting." Wilberforce answered politely.[39] When Darwin read Huxley's paper he congratulated him and called the paper a "complete and awful smasher . . . for Owen." As to Owen, he called Huxley a "humbug" for omitting the footnote on the similarity of man and apes in his Rede lecture to the "orthodox Cambridge dons."[40]

The second issue of the *Natural History Review* contained an article on an orang-utan brain by George Rolleston, who had won the chair of anatomy at Oxford, with Huxley's help over a candidate of Owen's. The article placed great emphasis on showing the cerebrum covering the cerebellum, and both a posterior horn and a hippocampus minor in orang-utan and human. It was illustrated with an elegant three-dimensional engraving of a horizontal dissection of the orang-utan brain showing a rather prominent hippocampus minor. (This same figure appeared again in the same issue, whether by accident or design, attached to an article entitled, "Crania of Ancient Races of Man." The figure was never cited in that article, which happened to contain another attack on Owen.) Rolleston noted that as he did not hold a materialist position, he believed the similarities of the brains of men and apes were, in any case, irrelevant to the species' mental status. (Huxley commented in a letter to Hooker that although Rolleston "had a great deal of Oxford slough [i.e., snake skin] to shed . . . his testimony on that very background has been of especial service."[41])

In the third issue, John Marshall, another friend of Huxley's, made essentially the same points about the falsity of Owen's three distinctions, in this case for the chimpanzee and with a great flourish of detailed measurements. Presumably to establish his credability, Marshall assures us to no "leaning toward any of the developmental hypotheses of the origin of species." He too explains that if a brain was not properly preserved and removed from the skull it would be grossly distorted and look like the one of a chimpanzee in Owen's paper. The article includes an actual mounted photographic print of a dissection showing the posterior horn and the hippocampus minor. A drawing based on this photograph was later published by Huxley and is shown in figure 4.3.[42]

The last issue of the year included an article on the anatomy of primate muscles, particularly those of the orang-utan, by W. S. Church.[43] The general theme was that examination of the range of variation among humans, particularly in the "lower" or "wild" races, reveals a smaller gap between the myology of humans and apes than noted by others, such as Owen. The author's dissections suggest that the chimpanzee and the gorilla "are able to point with their finger in the same manner as man."

Owen answered Huxley at a Royal Institution lecture reported in the *Athenaeum,* with a circulation of about 15,000, as compared with the *Review's* of about 1,000. Owen repeated his claim of the three structures specific to man, but hedged a little by saying that apes do not have a hippocampus minor "as defined in human anatomy." The accompanying brain illustrations were entitled "section of a Negro's brain" and "section of animal's brain." Both were otherwise unlabeled and their details unrecognizable and inaccurate. The next week Huxley wrote in to ridicule the inaccurate and unlabeled figures and to

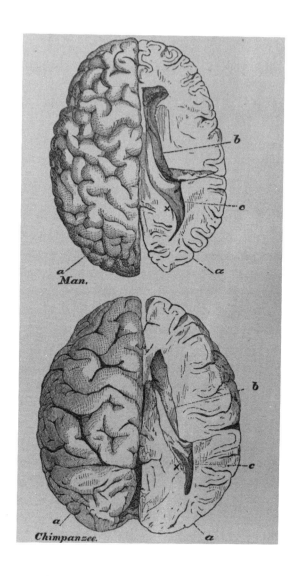

excoriate the reporter for failing to mention the numerous previous scientists who reported that the three critical structures were found in animals, since:

> doubtless Prof. Owen, following the course which would be taken
> by most men of science . . . allowed full weight to the affirmations
> of these eminent persons . . . and pointed out how they had been
> so misled as to describe . . . and figure . . . structures which have
> no existence.

In the following issue Owen blamed "the Artist" for the poor figures, but attested to the accuracy of the account otherwise. For a more accurate figure he referred the reader to his original paper, that is, to the distorted figure lifted from Schroeder van der Kolk and Vrolik.[44]

Owen's next detailed answer came in the *Annals and Magazine of Natural History* (circulation about 2,000). He republished both the Dutch chimpanzee figure (in spite of the comments of Gratiolet, Marshall, and Huxley) and Tiedemann's human brain figure that had been in his original paper, but he added drawings of the lateral ventricle in both species. The chimpanzee's ventricle had no hippocampus minor labeled on it, and Owen failed to mention that its source indicated one existed in this species. This time he cited the sources of his figures and pointed out that neither the Dutch nor German workers could have been influenced by their views on evolution since both had published before the *Origin* and even before *Vestiges*. He ended the paper by simply restating his three original claims for a difference between the brains of humans and all other creatures.[45]

Figure 4.3   "Drawings of the cerebral hemispheres of a Man and of a Chimpanzee of the same length, in order to show the relative proportions of the parts: the former taken from a specimen, which Mr. Flower, Conservator of the Museum of the Royal College of Surgeons, was good enough to dissect for me; the latter, from the photograph in Mr. Marshall's paper (Marshall, 1861) . . . *a,* posterior lobe; *b,* lateral ventricle; *c,* posterior cornu; *x,* the hippocampus minor" (Huxley, 1863).

Later that year Huxley weighed in with his own empirical paper "On the Brain of *Ateles paniscus*," the South American spider monkey, in the *Proceedings of the Zoological Society*. As with the other primate anatomy papers spurred by the controversy, the emphasis was on refuting Owen's three points, particularly on the hippocampus minor. The paper contained a set of carefully drawn human and simian coronal brain sections, as well as a horizontal dissection of the lateral ventricle, all designed to show prominently the hippocampus minor. In the course of his detailed study of this structure, Huxley corrected a major error in previous descriptions of human and other primate brains and effected a lasting change in sulcal terminology.

Before him, the major sulcus on the medical surface of the hemisphere was termed the hippocampal fissure and was supposed to extend from the corpus callosum to almost the posterior pole. In the course of studying sections through the hippocampus minor, Huxley realized that this hippocampal fissure consisted of two separate sulci, a posterior and anterior one. The indentation of the posterior one into the lateral ventricle formed the hippocampus minor, so he named it the calcarine sulcus after calcar avis. He named the anterior part the dentate sulcus, since it corresponded to the fascia dentata. "Calcarine sulcus," of course, entered into the permanent canon, but the term hippocampal fissure or sulcus was maintained for the anterior part (except by Huxley's followers), perhaps because the term dentate gyrus was already widespread.[46]

Huxley had only begun his campaign. In 1862 the onslaught against Owen spread to that most prestigious venue of them all, the *Philosophical Transactions of the Royal Society*. There another protégé of Huxley's, William Henry Flower, later Sir, after stating that he had no views on transmutation or the origin of man, proceeded to refute Owen's human-ape distinctions. He provided a detailed review of the earlier literature and then carefully presented the results of his own dissections of sixteen different primate species, including the orang-utan, several species of Old and New World monkeys, and several prosimians. Flower not only found a hippocampus minor in all these primates, but went on to claim that the hippocampus minor is largest in proportion to the mass of cerebral substance in the marmoset, next in monkeys, then apes,

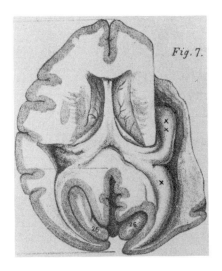
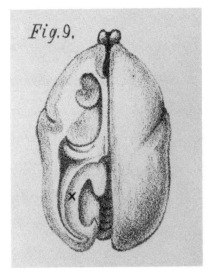

Figure 4.4 Horizontal views of the cerebrum of a vervet (left) and a marmoset (right).
"On the right side [of the vervet] the middle and posterior cornu are completely opened,
so as to exhibit the relative size and situation of the two hippocampi. In exposing the hippocampus minor to this extent, the limits of the cornu . . . have not been exceeded; but
as the walls are more or less adherent this must be regarded partly as a dissection. On the
left side the walls of the cornu remain undisturbed, part of the brain only having been cut
away to expose the commencement of the hippocampus major . . . " x, hippocampus major; xx, hippocampus minor (Flower, 1862).

and least in humans. Drawings of two of his dissections are shown in figure
4.4; the hippocampus minor in both, particularly the marmoset, certainly
appears prominent, if not rather exaggerated.

In addition to his being a close friend of Flower, Huxley's hand in the
paper is shown explicitly in two ways. First, the nomenclature that Flower used
included terms just introduced by Huxley. Second, Huxley was one of the
anonymous reviewers for Flower's paper and commented in his review "this
important paper should be published" (figure 4.5). The other reviewer was
John Marshall, another member of Huxley's anti-Owen team of
neuroanatomists.[47]

1862.

The Gov.t School of Mines & Cower
Urnigs or [illegible] April 4th 1862
by
Huxley

Before making my Report when
Mr Flower paper on the posterior
lober of the cerebrum in the Quadrumana
it is right that I should state
that the questions therein
discussed have been the subjects
g... controversy: that I have taken
an active part in that
controversy : & that Mr. Flower's
memoir contains a complete
confirmation of the statements
I have made

◆ ◆ ◆

Thomas H. Huxley

Huxley continued the campaign in the following year's *Natural History Review* with a long unsigned review of the leading French zoologist Geoffroy St. Hillaire's 1856 *Histoire Naturelle Generale,* quoting St. Hillaire at length on similarities of the brains of humans and apes, particularly[48]:

> for those of our readers who have followed the controversy respecting the brains of Apes and Man if that can be dignified by the name of a controversy where all the facts are on one side and mere empty assertion on the other.

When Schroeder van der Kolk and Vrolik discovered that Owen had repeatedly used the chimpanzee figure from their 1849 paper to justify his arguments they "resolved . . . to prevent the public from being misled." An

Figure 4.5   The beginning of Huxley's referee report on Flower's paper (1962), submitted to *Philosophical Transactions of the Royal Society,* which took Huxley's side in the controversy. The entire report (RR 4.97, Royal Society Archives) is as follows: "The Gov. School of Mines, Jermyn St. August 4, 1862. Before making my report upon Mr. Flower's paper 'On the posterior lobe of the cerebrum in the Quadrumana', it is right that I should state that the questions therein discussed have been the subjects of controversy: that I have taken an active part in that controversy: that Mr. Flower's memoir contains a complete confirmation of the statements I have made. This much premiered in order that the Committee of Papers may form their own judgement as to the extent to which my opinion is likely to be prejudiced, I may say, that both as regards manner and matter, Mr. Flower's memoir appears to me to be eminently worthy of a place in the Philosophical Transactions. Wisely avoiding even the appearance of entering into controversial discussions Mr. Flower has detailed with much clearness & precision of expression, a number of careful dissections—most of which have been made upon animals whose brains we possess, at present no sufficient account. The results of Mr. Flower's dissections of the Lemurine brains more particularly, are quite new & of very great importance. If it can be done without inconvenience I should recommend in the plates all the brains be drawn to the same absolute underlying length, as the variation in proportions become in this way far more obvious—Furthermore, as M. Gratiolet has already maintained the view that the Lemurs form a distinct subspecies—a reference should be added to this effect—to that part of Mr. Flower's paper which deals with this question. [signed] Thomas H. Huxley."

orang-utan had just died in the Amsterdam Zoo, so they dissected its brain. They reported at an 1862 meeting of the Dutch Royal Academy of Science that, in fact, this animal had an extensive posterior lobe covering the cerebellum as well as a posterior horn and a hippocampus minor. The attending audience, they wrote, recognized all three structures. The authors admitted the inadequacy of their original figure due to the way they had removed the brain from the cranium, and they disavowed any position on transmutation, but suggested that Owen had "gotten lost" and "fell into a trap" by his desire to combat Darwin. Huxley promptly reprinted the entire article, still in French, in his *Review.*[49]

That year and the next, the confrontations between Owen and Huxley continued in person and in print. For example, when Owen defended his position at the 1862 British Association meeting in Cambridge, his talk was reported in detail in the *Medical Times* and *Gazette* along with objections by Huxley and by his allies Rolleston and Flower, followed by Owen's rebuttal.[50] The next two issues contained further rounds between the combatants.

THE HIPPOCAMPUS MINOR GOES POP

While Owen and Huxley were fighting at meetings and in the scientific journals, the popular press was featuring and, usually, satirizing the hippocampus minor debate. One example is the anonymous poem from *Punch* shown in figure 4.6. It was written by Sir Philip Egerton, a paleontologist and member of parliament. After accurately epitomizing *Vestiges,* Darwin, and some recent archeological discoveries, the author focused in on Huxley and Owen's contest. In that year alone *Punch* had about a half dozen satirical pieces about the debate or its participants (figure 4.7).

Both Owen and Huxley and the hippocampus minor were featured in Charles Kingsley's children's fantasy *Water Babies,* originally published in 1863 and still in print and a favorite in Britain (see figure 4.1). At one point its child protagonist is puzzled at the strange things that are said at British Association

MONKEYANA.

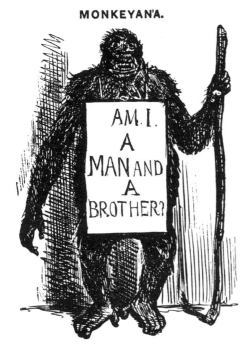

AM. I.
A
MAN AND
A
BROTHER?

Am I satyr or man?
    Pray tell me who can,
And settle my place in the scale.
    A man in ape's shape,
    An anthropoid ape,
Or monkey deprived of his tail?

The *Vestiges* taught,
    That all came from naught
By "development," so called, "progressive;"
    That insects and worms
    Assume higher forms
By modification excessive.

Then DARWIN set forth.
    In a book of much worth,
The importance of "Nature's selection;"
    How the struggle for life
    Is a laudable strife,
And results in "specific distinction."

Then HUXLEY and OWEN,
    With rivalry glowing,
With pen and ink rush to the scratch;
    'Tis Brain *versus* Brain,
    Till one of them's slain;
By Jove! it will be a good match!

Says OWEN, you can see
    The brain of Chimpanzee
Is always exceedingly small,
    With the hindermost "horn"
    Of extremity shorn,
And no "Hippocampus" at all.

The Professor then tells 'em
    That man's "cerebellum,"
From a vertical point you can't see;
    That each "convolution"
    Contains a solution,
Of "Archencephalic" degree.

Then apes have no nose,
    And thumbs for great toes,
And a pelvis both narrow and slight;
    They can't stand upright,
    Unless to show fight,
With "DU CHAILLU," that chivalrous knight!

Next HUXLEY replies,
    That OWEN he lies,
And garbles his Latin quotation;
    That his facts are not new,
    His mistakes not a few,
Detrimental to his reputation.

"To twice slay the slain,"
    By dint of the Brain,
(Thus HUXLEY concludes his review)
    Is but labour in vain,
    Unproductive of gain,
And so I shall bid you "Adieu!"

Zoological Gardens, May, 1861.   GORILLA

Figure 4.6   Part of a page from *Punch,* May 18, 1861. Several additional stanzas dealing with recent archeological discoveries are not shown. "Gorilla" here is the pseudonym for Sir Philip Egerton.

meetings. He had thought that the differences between him and an ape were such things as:

> being able to speak, and make machines, and know right from wrong, and say your prayers . . . rather than having . . . a hippopotamus major in your brain. He understands that . . . if a hippopotamus major is ever discovered in one single ape's brain, nothing will save your great-great-great-great-great-great-great-great-great-great-greater-greatest-grandmother from having been an ape too.

In an anonymous and well-informed eight-page squib entitled "A Report of a Sad Case Recently Tried before the Lord Mayor, Owen versus Huxley . . . " (figure 4.8), Owen and Huxley are dragged into court for brawling in the streets and disturbing the peace. The fight continues in court with much shouting of "posterior cornu," "hippocampus minor," and so on, as

> *Huxley:* Well, as I was saying, Owen and me is in the same trade; and we both cuts up monkeys, and I finds something in the brains of them. Hallo! says I, here's a hippocampus. No, there ain't says Owen. Look here says I. I can't see it he says and he sets to werriting and haggling about it, and goes and tells everybody, as what I finds ain't there, and what he finds is . . .

At the end of the trial, the Lord Mayor declines to punish either because "no punishment could reform offendors so incorrigible." He does suggest to Owen that rather than being bitter at being compared with an ape he might act less like one and more like a man. He suggests to Huxley that he is less interested in the truth than in destroying his rival.

Another anonymous pamphlet that year, entitled "Speech of Lord Dundreary . . . on the Great Hippocampus Questions," was also by Kingsley. The authors of these parodies not only knew every detail of the controversy but the personalities of the combatants and their friends intimately.

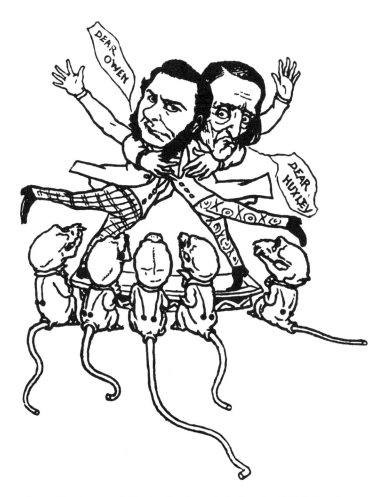

Figure 4.7 Owen and Huxley dancing a jig before the 1865 British Association Meeting. *Punch,* Sept. 23, 1865.

𝔄 𝔕𝔢𝔭𝔬𝔯𝔱

OF

A S A D C A S E,

Recently tried before the Lord Mayor,

OWEN *versus* HUXLEY,

In which will be found fully given the
Merits of the great Recent

B O N E C A S E

~~~~~~~~~~~~~~~~~

L O N D O N.
―――
1863.

G

―――

Evidence as to Man's Place in Nature

The School of Mines, Huxley's principal appointment for most of his life, sponsored an evening series of lectures for working men ("vouched for by their employers," although Karl Marx managed to attend). Huxley participated with great enthusiasm, writing that the working men:

> are as attentive and intelligent as the best audience I ever lectured to. In fact they *are* the best audience I ever had . . . I am sick of the dilettante middle classes.

As early as 1860 he began to devote these lectures to evolution and particularly to the evolution of man, a topic that Darwin avoided in public for another twenty years. On March 22, 1861, he wrote to his wife, "My working men stick by me wonderfully, the house being fuller than ever last night. By next Friday evening they will all be convinced that they are monkeys . . . "[51] Soon Huxley expanded these lectures into a book telling Sir Charles Lyell,

> I mean to give the whole history of the [Owen] business . . . so that the paraphrase of Sir Ph. Egerton's line "To which Huxley replies that Owen he lies," shall be unmistakable. [See figure 4.6.]

The book, designed for a lay audience, was *Evidence as to Man's Place in Nature*. Darwin loved it, exclaiming: "Hurrah the monkey book has come." It was enormously successful, selling out at once and quickly going through several more printings.[52]

The first part, "On the Natural History of the Man-like Apes," is largely a review of travelers' accounts of various apes, stressing their humanlike intel-

Figure 4.8   Title page of an eight-page squib anonymously published and written by G. Pycroft. In it Owen and Huxley are dragged into court for brawling in the streets over the hippocampus minor and related matters.

167

ligence, emotions, and social life. It thus lays the basis for Darwin and Romanes's florid anthropomorphizing in defense of psychological continuity between humans and animals. When this tendency to attribute high mental functions to animals was reduced by C. Lloyd Morgan's law of parsimony, Occam's razor for students of animal behavior, this continuity argument became the basis of modern behavioristic psychology.[53]

The second part, "On the Relations of Man to the Lower Animals," is the heart of the book. It begins with arguments from embryology and cell theory for the fundamental unity of all animals, including, of course, humans. Then the bones, skull, and teeth of humans and apes are discussed, with the conclusion that "the lower Apes and the Gorilla . . . differ more than the Gorilla and the Man." Next, and it almost seems like the raison d'etre for the whole book, we come to an account of the fundamental similarity of the brain of apes and humans, particularly the possession by both of a posterior lobe, a posterior horn, and a hippocampus minor. The account is a twelve-page, step-by-step argument, but perhaps it had to be since the audience addressed had never heard of a brain ventricle, let alone the hippocampus minor. At the end of the chapter, Huxley points out that the close similarity of human and ape that he has just demonstrated proves the validity of Linnaeus's original Primate order, and ends by stating, in a rather offhand manner, that Darwin's theory provides an explanation of the origin of man from ape.

Interposed between the second and third parts are six pages of fine print providing, "a succinct History of the Controversy respecting the Cerebral Structure of Man and the Apes," that is, how Owen "suppressed" and denied the truth about the hippocampus minor, posterior horn, and posterior lobe, and how this was now a matter of "personal veracity." The final portion of *Man's Place,* "On Some Fossil Remains of Man," deals with the evidence for a fossil link between ape and human, which Huxley admitted was very meager indeed.

At the time, judging by a sample of the reviews, Huxley's book was regarded chiefly as a polemic against Owen, favorably by Huxley's partisans who were in the majority by now, and unfavorably by Owen's allies. Darwin, natural selection, and even evolution, as distinct from the human's systematic status, are not major issues in these reviews and indeed they are not major concerns in the book. Probably the most influential evaluation was that of Sir Charles Lyell, Britain's leading geologist and one of its most eminent scientists. Through nine editions his *Principles of Geology* rejected the idea of evolution. Now in *Antiquity of Man* he evenhandedly discussed the pros and cons of Darwin's theory, disappointing Darwin, but actually moving a very long way closer to him. He also reviewed the hippocampus minor debate in detail. Lyell came down totally and unambiguously on Huxley's side, which must have effectively ended the discussion in the scientific community.[54]

Owen, no surprise, attempted to refute Lyell and continued to defend his classification scheme against its critics. He even found a new support for the importance of the hippocampus minor: that it was absent, or virtually so, in an "idiot."[55]

Owen's final statements on the controversy are in *On the Anatomy of Vertebrates*. There his brain figures are accurate, and in a long footnote he finally admits, citing himself as well as the earlier literature, that in apes "all the homologous parts of the human cerebral organ exist." However, this admission, he believes, does not invalidate or even threaten his classification of man in a separate subclass because the critical structures, the posterior lobe, the posterior horn, and the hippocampus minor, exist in apes only ". . . under modified form and low grades of development." As to Huxley and his neuroanatomical allies, their attacks on his classificatory scheme were "puerile," "ridiculous," and "disgraceful."[56]

Owen's original aim was to define the uniqueness of humankind, to find an objective way of differentiating humans from animals that was (a) qualitative and not merely quantitative, (b) solidly grounded in anatomical science rather than theology or speculation, and (c) based on the brain, the origin of the most striking differences between humans and animals. His downfall was not this goal but his hubris in stubbornly defending his errors in trying to reach it. The tragedy was classic: Owen fell from the pinnacle of British science to be remembered, when at all, for his obstinate errors in this debate, rather than for his real contributions.

THE SOURCES OF OWEN'S THREE CRITERIA

Where did Owen get his three benchmarks whose repudiation by Huxley destroyed his credibility as a critic of Darwin and evolution? One source for his idea that the posterior extent of the cerebrum in humans was a powerful indicator of their elevated taxonomic status was probably a figure in Fletcher's *Rudiments of Physiology*. This figure shows a series of dorsal views of the brain, drawn to the same size, starting with cuttlefish [sic], then eel, turtle, bird, marmot, and "up" through otter, to orang-utan, to the human.[57] A line is drawn at the posterior border of the cerebrum (or its supposed homolog) to show that moving "upward" in the animal scale the cerebrum moves posteriorly until, in the human, it covers the rest of the brain, the cerebellum being the last structure to disappear from view. Fletcher's idea of these systematic changes correlating with increasing complexity was used by Chambers as a major argument for evolution in *Vestiges* and therefore must have been well known to Owen, at least through this source (Owen had originally been quite sympathetic to *Vestiges*[58]). As mentioned previously, this idea that the cerebellum was exposed even in the highest nonhuman primates was supported by published drawings of "distorted" ape brains.[59]

Owen's choice of structures in the lateral ventricles for his other two ways of distinguishing humans and animals appears to be a persistence of the importance Galen gave the ventricles centuries earlier. The ventricles played a central role in his physiological system, a set of theoretical views that dominated Western medicine for over 1,400 years and was influential into the nineteenth century. Galen thought the ventricles were the primary site of production of psychic pneuma, which he believed was a critical mediator of cerebral function and the medium of transmission in sensory and motor nerves. The early church fathers, particularly Nemesius, Bishop of Emesia (fourth century), radically altered Galen's conceptions of the structure and function of the ventricles, transforming the ventricles into three more "perfect" spheres. Galen had localized sensory and motor functions in the solid portions of the cerebrum, the former anteriorly and the latter posteriorly. The church fathers, however, were looking for a less mundane site for the interaction of the body and soul and chose for this purpose the "empty" spaces in the brain that Galen described, the ventricles. They then took the Aristotelian faculties of the mind, sensation, cognition, and memory, and located them in the anterior, middle, and posterior ventricles, respectively (see figure 1.7). Drawings of this ventricular localization of mental function hardly changed for over a thousand years except for the expressions on the faces.

When systematic brain dissection began again in the Renaissance the brains were usually dissected from the top down, often in situ. The ventricles were carefully depicted and labeled because of their importance in Galenic theory. The most famous of these early horizontal dissections was that of Vesalius in his revolutionary work, *On the Fabric of the Human Body,* published in 1543 (see figure 1.10). Horizontal views in which the ventricular features are prominent continued to be a common way of depicting the internal structure of the human brain into the nineteenth century (see figure 1.15). Thus, ventricular structures were carefully depicted and named, whereas the cortex was often drawn in a schematic fashion, since, until Gall and phrenology, it was usually thought to be unimportant. The theoretical importance of the ventricles persisted presumably because no better theory of brain function emerged, and better theories, not better facts, are required to overturn a theory. Given this tradition it is not all that surprising that Owen, looking for important and "higher" parts of the human brain, looked into the ventricles. See chapter 1 for further discussion of ventricular theory.

MAN'S PLACE IN NATURE IN HISTORY

A second edition of Huxley's *Man's Place in Nature* was published in 1896. A number of things had changed since the first edition. The general idea of evolution, including that of humans, was now accepted by most of the scientific community. Darwin's *The Descent of Man* had been published offering detailed mechanisms for the evolution of the human body, mind, and morals. It contained an appendix by Huxley on the similarities and differences between human and ape brains. The hippocampus minor is mentioned only in passing, but never Owen. Sir Richard had died in 1892 and in the ultimate confirmation of the saying, "history is written by the victors," his grandson asked Huxley for an account of Owen's "Position in the History of Anatomical Science" to include in the book he was writing on the life of Owen.[60] Huxley gave him sixty pages that did not refer to any of their bitter disputes and were full of phrases such as "unabated industry," "wide knowledge," "great service," "splendid record," and "sagacious interpretations." By this time Huxley was the Right Honorable (a privy counselor) and had been president of the Royal, Ethnological, Geological, and Palaeontographical Societies, the British Association, and the National Association of Science Teachers, as well as university president and dean.

More generally, the social and political scene had changed. The Reform Act of 1867 giving the urban working class the vote eliminated the threat of revolution, or perhaps the decline of this threat made the Act possible, and the end of religious tests had opened the doors of Oxford and Cambridge to dissenters and Jews as students and faculty. Both developments tended to reduce the political charge of evolutionary ideas. The dominance of the Oxbridge clergyman-naturalist had given way to that of the professional scientist of which Huxley was the archetype. As much as personality clashes or scientific differences, the conflict between Owen and Huxley represented this transfer of power. Although they came from similar middle-class, nonuniversity backgrounds, Owen early attached himself to the medical, religious, and political establishment. In contrast, Huxley fought to professionalize science and free it from the dominance of clergy and gentry, although he carefully kept his distance from the political radicals of the time.[61] In defeating Owen and his backers, Huxley and his friends had become the Establishment, and in doing so, the hippocampus minor was Huxley's most successful weapon.

The new edition of *Man's Place* reflected changes in the status of evolutionary theory and of Huxley himself. The title had become more assertive, dropping *"Evidence as to"* and becoming simply *Man's Place in Nature*. The section "Succinct History" of Owen's supposed perfidy was eliminated entirely and Owen hardly mentioned at all.

Today this book is usually viewed as a triumph of evolutionary thought rather than an attack on Owen or a defense of Linnaeus, and its relevance to the hippocampus minor has been totally lost. Huxley is admired for charging in where Darwin feared to tread for another eight years. Homer Smith, physiologist and historian of science, called it "the first . . . [and still] . . . definitive statement of the naturalistic interpretation [of man] . . . ," Sir Arthur Keith, pioneering anthropologist, claimed it "laid the basis for a true science of anthropology" and "can only be compared to Harvey's *Movement of the Heart and Blood*." Ashley Montagu, in an introduction to a paperback edition, called it a "great classic of science" and "among the most inspiring."[62]

The Place of the Hippocampus Minor in Man's Search for Meaning

Richard Owen identified the hippocampus minor and its associated structures as the touchstone of humanness. Other choices for this function from brain anatomy have included the size of the frontal lobes, brain laterality, and the position of the lunate sulcus. Perhaps the earliest was that of Herophilus, the Alexandrian anatomist in the second century BCE who attributed man's greater intelligence to his more complex cerebellum, or so Galen, in ridiculing this view, tells us.[63]

Thomas Huxley chose language in *Man's Place* as the criterion of humanity, and some of its contemporary reviewers pointed out that in doing so he was playing the same game he attacked when Owen played it.[64] Human language continues to be a popular candidate for a hippocampus minor, although whether the uniqueness of language lies in its unbounded vocabulary, infinite set of sentences of arbitrary size and complexity, ability to code distant time and place, self-reference, or ability to lie is unclear.

For his ordering of organisms, Linnaeus preferred sexual characteristics, at least for plants, and when he could get them, for animals (e.g., mammae).

Perhaps inspired by him, variety of coital positions, desire for privacy during intercourse, and orgasm in females have all been offered as distinguishing features of *Homo sapiens* (and counterindicated), as has the ratio of the size of the erect penis and of the female breasts to body weight.[65] DNA was a transient hope, but the difference between human and chimpanzee (about 1.6%) is rather anxiety provoking.

One basic human characteristic does seem to be the need to establish differences between ourselves and our closest relatives; for that purpose, the hippocampus minor may be as good a criterion as any other.[66]

NOTES

1. Lamarck, 1809; Mayr, 1982; Desmond, 1989.

2. The fear and reality of persecution for unorthodox views in Victorian biology was virtually ignored until Gruber (1974) showed it to be the major cause of Darwin's delay in publishing. Gruber's insights may have been related to his own political persecution during the McCarthy era in the United States. Desmond and Moore (1992) also make fear of persecution an important theme in Darwin's life.

3. Chambers is treated in detail by Secord (1989), Desmond (1992), Ruse (1979), and Mayr (1982). The first (1844) edition of *Vestiges* was reprinted (1969) by Leicester University Press. Chambers published ten more editions, many of which were responsive to the detailed criticisms of his reviewers. The twelfth (1884) posthumous edition finally named its author, common knowledge by then.

4. Sedgwick, 1850. The quotations were found by Young (1970a), Mayr (1982), and Desmond (1992).

5. Huxley, 1854. Huxley later called this "the only review I ever had qualms of conscience about, on the grounds of needless savagery," (L. Huxley, 1900).

6. Disraeli, 1847.

7. Desmond, 1992; Young, 1970a, 1973.

8. Mayr, 1982; Darwin, 1909; Wallace, 1905; F. Darwin, 1887.

9. Ritvo, 1987.

10. Owen (1894). Upper crust social events are scattered throughout these two volumes by Owen's grandson, but there is very little about the course of Owen's rich scientific life and correspondence.

11. E.g., Owen, 1853, 1855.

12. Owen, 1858, 1859.

13. Indeed, as demonstrated by Gould (1981), their measurements of crania and brains tended to confirm their prior beliefs. An interesting exception was Wallace (1891), who stated in *Natural Selection* that the "brain of the lowest savage . . . is little inferior to that of the highest types of man"; and in *My Life,* (1905), "The more I see of uncivilized people, the better I think of human nature and the essential differences between civilized and savage men seem to disappear." Wallace's tolerant and relatively nonracist attitude may have been the result of having lived among Pacific Islanders for eight years and traveled under their care on long voyages over the open seas. In contrast, Darwin and Huxley made their observations about the primitive minds of the lower races largely from the decks of *H.M.S. Beagle* and *H.M.S. Rattlesnake.* Wallace's views of the full development of the brain and in some cases the moral sense among "savages" led him to reject totally natural selection as a basis for humans' intellectual and moral development (Wallace, 1891). He appealed to "some higher intelligence" as an alternative. The fact that such religious mysticism was now out of fashion, plus his involvement in various spiritualist activities such as table rapping, obscured Wallace's observations and insights of how cultural evolution was replacing biological evolution in the development of human civilization (Eiseley, 1961). Otherwise, perhaps a "social Wallacism" might have developed.

14. Gould, 1981; Tiedemann, 1836; Topinard, 1878. Schiebinger's (1993) detailed discussion of Baartman has a valuable set of references to the primary and secondary literature. The results of Cuvier's dissection of Baartman's genitals are in the Musee de l'Homme in Paris (Gould, 1982, a gem). Huxley (1861a) commented that she "had the honor of being anatomized by Cuvier."

15. Burkhardt and Smith, 1985, vol. VI.

16. Lewis, 1923; Meyer, 1971.

17. Kingsley, 1863.

18. See chapter 1; Young, 1970b.

19. The state of knowledge of the brain in the nineteenth century is dealt with in more detail in chapter 1; Young, 1970b; Boring, 1950.

20. Mitchell, 1901; L. Huxley, 1900; Desmond, 1984.

21. Letter to his friend and predecessor at the School of Mines, Edward Forbes (Desmond, 1984).

22. Letter to W. Macleay, an entomologist he had met in Sydney, describing the British scientific scene (L. Huxley, 1900; Desmond, 1984).

23. Bibby (1959) has a synoptic curriculum vitae of Huxley. Some of the scientific attacks: by Huxley on Owen, "Observations upon the Anatomy and Physiology of Salpa and Pyrosoma" (1851); "Contributions to the Anatomy of Brachiopoda" (1854–1855); "Lectures on General Natural History" (1856a); "Owen and R. Jones on Comparative Anatomy" (1856b); "Vestiges of the Natural History of Creation" (1854); and "On the Theory of the Vertebrate Skull" (1859). Owen's treatise was *The Archetype and Homologies of the Vertebrate Skeleton,* London (1848). For naturphilosophie and its influence on Owen, see Nordenskiold (1928) and MacLeod (1965).

24. Owen, 1894.

25. Huxley's letter to the Medical Directory is quoted in DiGregorio (1984); Huxley's letter to a friend (F. Dyster) is quoted in Desmond (1984). The record seems to show that Owen was appointed lecturer at the School of Mines for these lectures; and Huxley's title there was also lecturer, not professor. Both individuals at the time probably considered they were entitled to call themselves professor since Owen had just held a chair at the Royal College of Surgeons and Huxley had a temporary one at the Royal Institute.

26. The X Club was a dining club of Huxley and about eight of his friends devoted to "science, pure and free, untrammelled by religious dogma." It included botanist J. D. Hooker, physicist J. Tyndall, ethologist J. Lubbock, and philosopher Herbert Spencer. It gradually accrued enormous power in British science. Its influence ranged from membership, medals, and offices in the Royal Society and on journal editorial boards to the standards for science teachers and school science curricula. See Barton (1990), Desmond (1984), and Jensen (1991) including its rich notes.

27. Burkhardt and Smith, 1985, vol. VII; L. Huxley, 1900; Mayr, 1982; Ruse, 1979.

28. L. Huxley, 1990; Ellegard, 1958; F. Darwin, 1887.

29. *Athenaeum,* July 7, 1860; L. Huxley, 1900.

30. L. Huxley, 1900.

31. *Athenaeum,* July 14, 1860; L. Huxley, 1900; F. Darwin, 1887, 1903; Jensen, 1991 who provides the sources for all the contemporary or quasi-contemporary quotations cited here; see also Gould (1986). Comparison with Waterloo is Moore's (1979); "murder and martyrdom" is Irvine's (1955).

32. Both were Huxley's self-descriptions (L. Huxley, 1900).

33. Huxley, 1896; L. Huxley, 1900; Desmond, 1984. Characteristically, Darwin told Huxley that the *Review* was a waste of time and he should get on with his own original research instead (F. Darwin, 1903).

34. Huxley, 1861a; Desmond, 1984.

35. Owen, 1835.

36. Tiedemann, 1821, 1827, 1836.

37. Schroeder van der Kolk and Vrolik (1849).

38. Tiedemann, 1821, 1827, 1836.

39. Blinderman, 1957.

40. F. Darwin, 1903.

41. Rolleston, 1861; L. Huxley, 1900.

42. Marshall, 1861; Huxley, 1863.

43. Church, 1861.

44. These exchanges are in the *Athenaeum* between Mar. 23, 1861 and Apr. 13, 1861. The circulation figures are from Ellegard (1958).

45. Owen, 1861.

46. Huxley, 1861b; Meyer, 1971.

47. Flower, 1862. The reviews are available in the *Archives of the Royal Society,* RR.96-7 (Huxley's reviews) and RR.4.95,98 (Marshall's reviews).

48. [Huxley], 1862.

49. Lyell, 1863; Schroeder van der Kolk and Vrolik, 1862.

50. October 11, 1962.

51. Bibby, 1959; L. Huxley, 1900.

52. L. Huxley, 1900; F. Darwin, 1903; Blinderman, 1971; Desmond and Moore, 1992.

53. Darwin, 1871; Romanes, 1882; Morgan, 1894; Boring, 1950; Boakes, 1984.

54. Blake, 1863; DiGregorio, 1984; Lyell, 1863; F. Darwin, 1903.

55. Owen, 1863a, b.

56. Owen, 1866.

57. Fletcher, 1835; Secord, 1989.

58. MacLeod, 1965; Richards, 1987.

59. Schroeder van der Kolk and Vrolik, 1849; Tiedemann, 1836.

60. Owen, 1894.

61. Desmond, 1984.

62. Smith, 1955; Keith, 1925; Montagu, 1959.

63. Galen, 1968.

64. E.g., [Anonymous], 1863.

65. Diamond, 1992.

---

66. The Darwin industry grinds on. Since this chapter was written, three major biographies of the principals have appeared: Brown (1995) on Darwin, Desmond (1994) on Huxley, and Rupke (1994) on Owen. Rupke's sympathetic treatment of Owen maintains that Owen's desire for a Natural History museum over the opposition of Huxley was a major source of their quarrels about evolution.

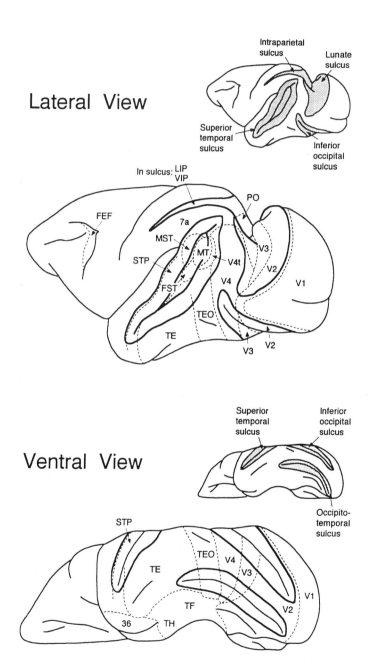

BEYOND STRIATE CORTEX: HOW LARGE PORTIONS OF THE
TEMPORAL AND PARIETAL CORTEX BECAME VISUAL AREAS

How does the pattern of energy falling on the retina yield the complexity of our visual experience and the richness of our visual memory? How do we recognize flowers and faces and all the other infinitely varied inhabitants of our visual world? How do we know where objects around us are located even when our eyes, head, and bodies and the objects themselves are moving? At midtwentieth century, the answer to these questions seemed clear: striate cortex (area 17), and only striate cortex, was responsible for the visual perception of form, color, movement, and space—for our consciousness of the visual world. As Karl Lashley, professor of neuropsychology at Harvard and the leading physiological psychologist of the day, put it, " . . . visual habits are dependent upon the striate cortex and upon no other part of the cerebral cortex."[1] The leading textbook concurred[2]:

Figure 5.1   Lateral and ventral views of a macaque monkey brain illustrating some of the known subdivisions of visual cortex. In each of the smaller drawings, the shaded areas correspond to sulci that have been opened up to show the areas located within them. FEF, frontal eye field; FST, fundus of the superior temporal sulcus visual area; TE and TEO, cytoarchitectonic areas of inferior temporal cortex; MST, medial superior temporal area; PO, parieto-occipital visual area; STP, superior temporal polysensory area; TF and TH, cytoarchitectonic areas of the parahippocampal cortex; 36, cytoarchitectonic area 36 of perirhinal cortex; V1, striate cortex or area 17; V2, V3, V4, second, third, and fourth visual areas; V4t, transitional V4 area (after Gross et al., 1993).

In human subjects there is no evidence that any area of the cortex other than the visual area 17 is important in the primary capacity to see patterns . . . Whenever the question has been tested in animals the story has been the same.

As recently as 1975, Krieg's monumental treatise on primate brain anatomy asserted that "image formation and recognition is all in area 17 and is entirely intrinsic . . . the connections of area 17 are minimal."[3]

Today, we know that an area much larger than striate cortex is involved in visual function. Specifically, the boundaries of the cortical region involved in visual function have flowed forward out of the occipital lobe, deep into the temporal, parietal, and even frontal lobes; visual cortex consists of more than two dozen discrete visual areas making up more than half the primate cerebral cortex (figure 5.1).

In this chapter I first consider the discovery of the visual areas adjacent to striate cortex in the occipital lobe and then the discovery of visual cortex in the temporal and parietal lobes. Our survey ends in 1982 with the introduction of the idea of two cortical streams of visual processing.

SENSORY CENTERS IN THE CEREBRAL CORTEX

The modern study of the cerebral cortex began in the latter half of the nineteenth century, a period Hans-Lukas Teuber called the heroic age of neuropsychology.[4] The tasks faced were Herculean, the principal players with their bushy beards and fierce countenances were larger than life, and the virulence of their clashes went well beyond the usual academic disputes.

A central question in this period was the localization of discrete sensory centers in the cerebral cortex. The idea that the cortex consisted of a set of organs with specific psychological functions was first systematically proposed by Franz Joseph Gall in his phrenological system at the beginning of the century.[5] The possibility of the localization of psychological function was actively debated until 1861, when Paul Broca's demonstration of a language center in the frontal lobe was viewed as ending the debate in Gall's favor.[6] Further support for Gall's general idea came from Gustav Fritsch and Edouard Hitzig's discovery of motor cortex.[7] As described in chapter 1, a major controversy concerned the location of the visual center: David Ferrier placed it in the angular gyrus of the parietal lobe, whereas E. A. Schäfer and then Hermann Munk claimed it was in the occipital lobe. By the turn of the century, the visual area was firmly placed in occipital cortex and soon after identified with striate cortex. Ever since then, as recounted in the rest of this chapter, visual mechanisms have been discovered in the cerebral cortex outside of striate cortex.

VISUAL ASSOCIATION CORTEX

In the last decades of the nineteenth century Paul Flechsig,[8] on the basis of time of myelination, divided the cerebral cortex into three regions: the primary or projection zones, the intermediate zones, and the terminal zones, the latter two together called the association cortex (see figure 1.24). He chose the term "association" because he believed that these regions myelinated in humans at the age when children began to associate the different senses with each other and with movement. In his scheme, only the primary areas received sensory input from below the cortex, and this input was confined to one modality. The output of the modality-specific primary areas was to the intermediate zones surrounding each of the primary areas; they remained unimodal and further elaborated the sensations into perceptions, which might then be "associated" with the other sensory modalities by way of long association fibers in the terminal zone. At this time psychology was dominated by British associationism (typified by John Stuart Mill and Alexander Bain), and association cortex was quickly assigned the tasks of the "association of sensations into perceptions, images, ideas and memories."[9] The idea that sensations were fundamentally different from perceptions was much older, deriving from Aristotle, as in his dictum, "It is not the bell that enters the ear, but the energy of the sound that leaves the bell." This difference was emphasized by David Hume in the eighteenth century in his distinction between "impressions and ideas," and in the twentieth century by E. B. Titchener.[10] Flechsig's concept that each sensory receiving area had an adjacent modality-specific association area persisted into the early 1940s as shown in figure 5.2, taken from the leading physiological psychology text book of the day.

At the turn of the twentieth century, inspired by these theoretical conceptions, the intermediate visual zone was termed "visuopsychic" to distinguish it from the primary visual or visuosensory area now identified with striate cortex. On "histological" grounds, J. S. Bolton and Alfred Campbell, both working in the Rainhill Asylum, Lancashire, defined the visuopsychic area as a 1.3- to 2-cm strip surrounding the visuosensory area. As the latter put it, the visuosensory center is "a primary station . . . for the receipt of impressions derived from . . . both retinal fields." In contrast, the visuopsychic center, ". . . is an area wherein visual impressions are further dealt with in the process of elaboration and intellectual interpretations . . ."[11] The arguments for the functions attributed to the visuopsychic area as opposed to the visuosensory one were strictly anatomical, embryological, and theoretical: Campbell was pessimistic about the possibility of finding patients with sufficiently discrete lesions to distinguish the two areas.

G. Elliot Smith, professor of anatomy at the Egyptian School of Medicine in Cairo, divided the Bolton-Campbell visuopsychic area into a zone adjacent to striate cortex, which he named parastriate cortex, and an outer zone, which he named peristriate cortex.[12] These areas corresponded roughly to Brodmann's areas 18 and 19, designated at about the same time, and to the ones von Economo (1929) named areas OB and OA in 1929.[13] The outer zone, peristriate or 19, was assumed to have more complex psychic functions than the inner zone, parastriate or 18 (figure 5.3). Collectively, areas 18 and 19 were often grouped as visual association cortex, which together with temporal and parietal association cortex was known as posterior association cortex.

With assumption and theory continuing to outstrip evidence, psychic blindness, or, as it came to be known, visual agnosia, was believed to be caused by "loss of associations between optical sensations and what they signify," as

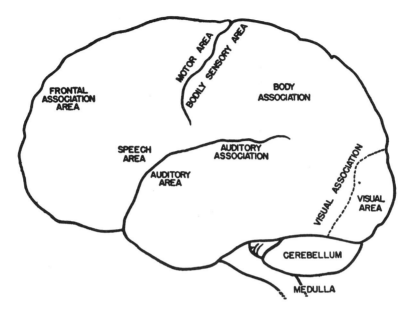

Figure 5.2   Side view of the human cerebral cortex showing how each sensory area was believed to have an adjacent association area devoted to the corresponding sense (Morgan, 1943).

William James put it.[14] Therefore it was assumed to be due to damage to the visuopsychic areas. As additional cases of visual agnosia were reported they were usually attributed to damage to this visual association cortex, although the evidence was rarely enough to justify more than a vague posterior location of the injury, if that.

Originally, it had been thought that only striate cortex was a cortical retina, that is, topographically organized with a "map" of the retina; parastriate and peristriate cortex (areas 18 and 19) were not believed to be topographically organized. Rather, they were supposed to be concerned with perceptual and association functions and not sensory function. With the rise of electrical mapping of sensory cortex, however, quite the contrary soon became clear.

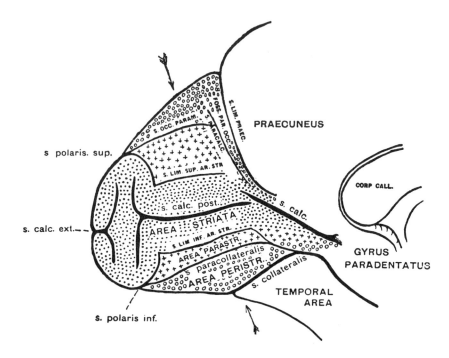

Figure 5.3 Elliot Smith's (1907) "Diagram to illustrate the distribution of the cortical areas on the mesial surface of the occipital region of the left hemisphere." He was the first to use the designations area striata, area parastriata, and area peristriata.

In the 1940s, using evoked responses recorded with large surface electrodes in the cat, S. A. Talbot and Wade Marshall found a second topographically organized visual area immediately adjacent to striate cortex, coextensive with area 18.[15] Then, in 1965 Hubel and Wiesel, using microelectrode recording of single-neuron activity in the cat, confirmed the second visual area, now called V2, and found an adjacent third retinotopically organized visual area, V3.[16] So the original cortical retina or map in striate cortex turned out to be surrounded by two other cortical retinas. As we will see later, in both the cat and the monkey, many more cortical retinas—maps of the retina—were found.

A Lost Observation on Temporal Cortex

In the nineteenth-century welter and confusion over the location of the visual and other sensory centers, two important observations were lost (or ignored) and had to be rediscovered decades later. The first was on temporal lobe damage. When this observation was eventually repeated and extended, it led to the discovery of the critical role of inferior temporal neurons in object recognition. The second observation was on parietal lobe damage. It led to the realization of the critical role of posterior parietal cortex in spatial vision.

The first observation was made by Brown and Schäfer in 1888 in an article that played a definitive role in establishing the visual area in the occipital lobes.[17] Brown and Schäfer opposed Ferrier's views not only on the location of the visual area but also on localization of the auditory area in the superior temporal gyrus. One of their strongest pieces of evidence against an auditory center in the temporal lobe was their monkey known as the "Tame One," who had received large bilateral temporal lobe lesions (figure 5.4). This animal was demonstrated at several international meetings and its lack of deafness was attested to by an examining committee at the 1887 meeting of the Neurological Society. More relevant to our story than this absence of deafness were the striking changes in postoperative behavior that Brown and Schäfer described:

A remarkable change is manifested in the disposition of the Monkey. Prior to the operations he was very wild and even fierce, assaulting any person who teased or tried to handle him. Now, he voluntarily approaches all persons indifferently, allows himself to be handled, or even to be teased or slapped without making any attempt at retaliation or endeavoring to escape. His memory and intelligence seem deficient. He gives evidence of hearing, seeing and of his senses generally, but *it is clear that he no longer clearly understands the meanings of the sights, sounds and other impressions that reach him* [my italics]. Every object he endeavors to feel, taste and

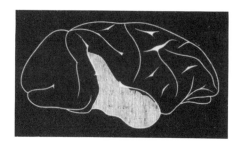

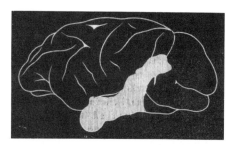

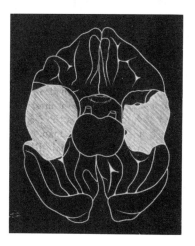

Figure 5.4   Temporal lobectomy in Brown and Schäfer's 1888 study that produced a strange set of symptoms later rediscovered as the Klüver-Bucy syndrome (Schäfer, 1888a).

smell, and to carefully examine. This is the case not only with inanimate objects, but also with persons and with his fellow Monkeys. And even after having examined an object in this way with the utmost care and deliberation, he will, on again coming across the same object accidentally even a few minutes afterwards, go through exactly the same process, as if he had forgotten his previous experiments. He appears no longer to discriminate between the different kinds of food e.g., he no longer picks out the currants from a dish of food but devours everything just as it happens to come. He still however possesses the sense of taste, for when given a raisin which has been partially filled with quinine he shows evident signs of distaste, and refuses to eat the fruit. . .

The authors concluded that

On localization of functions the experiment throws no direct light . . . a general depression of the intellectual faculties has resulted and a condition resembling idiocy produced.

Schäfer described his findings on the visual and auditory cortical areas in several further publications and repeatedly used this animal's normal hearing as an argument against the existence of a temporal lobe auditory center. However, he never again mentioned the strange effects of removal of the temporal lobes except to say that it produced "idiocy."[18] Given the disputes over the location of the basic cortical sensory areas and the fact that even Schäfer himself never referred again to the effects of temporal lobe removal, it is not surprising that these observations were lost. They were rediscovered only ten years after they were repeated by two Chicago Scientists, Klüver and Bucy.

THE KLÜVER-BUCY SYNDROME

Heinrich Klüver was a professor at the University of Chicago for over fifty years and was responsible for the development of many of the modern techniques for studying visual cognition in monkeys.[19] He was also quite interested in the effects of mescaline on perception, particularly on himself, and wrote a little book called *Mescal, the Divine Plant.*[20] Klüver thought that the hallucinations or aura that sometimes precede a temporal lobe seizure resembled a mescaline-induced hallucination, and on that basis he speculated that the temporal lobes might be the site of action of mescaline. To test this possibility he arranged for the neurosurgeon Paul Bucy to remove the temporal lobes of several monkeys to see whether, postoperatively, mescaline still induced behaviors suggesting mescaline hallucination.[21]

The effects of mescaline seem to have been the same after the temporal lobe removals as before, but the undrugged temporal lobectomized monkeys showed a strange and intriguing set of behavioral changes. This set of symptoms became known as the Klüver-Bucy syndrome. Klüver summarized them as follows[22]:

1. . . . [P]sychic blindness or visual agnosia . . . the ability to recognize and detect the meaning of objects on visual criteria alone seems to be lost although the animal exhibits no or at least no gross defects in the ability to discriminate visually.

2. . . . [S]trong oral tendencies in the sense that the monkey insists on examining all objects by mouth.

3. There is an excessive tendency to attend and react to every visual stimulus.

4. . . . [P]rofound changes in emotional behavior, and there may even be a complete loss of emotional responses in the sense that . . . anger and fear are not exhibited. All expressions of emotions . . . may be completely lost.

5. . . . [S]triking increase in the amount and diversity of sexual behavior. It exhibits forms of autosexual, heterosexual and homosexual behavior rarely or never seen in normal monkeys.

6. . . . [A] remarkable change in dietary habits . . . [particularly]
. . . a tendency to consume large quantities of . . . [meat].

Ten years after his original study, Klüver came upon the 1881 Brown and Schäfer paper with the description of the monkey with the bilateral temporal lobectomy, and wrote:

> It is evident that the observations of Brown and Schäfer agree fully with ours, particularly with reference to the picture of psychic blindness, the oral tendencies, the "hypermetamorphosis" and the striking changes in emotional behavior. It is evident that the bilateral lesions . . . were comparable in extent to the lesions produced in our experimental animals.

Klüver and Bucy had reported that they could not produce their syndrome or any of its components by lesions smaller than ones of both temporal lobes, and suggested that the syndrome was a unitary one that could not be "fractionated." However, about ten years later that is exactly what began to happen.

FRACTIONATION OF THE KLÜVER-BUCY SYNDROME

By the 1920s, with the fall of association psychology and the rise of Gestalt psychology, the pendulum began to swing away from cortical localization of all but primary sensory and motor functions and toward the antilocalizationist views in the earlier holistic tradition of Friedrich Goltz and Jacques Loeb.[23] Attacks on the association of visual agnosia with damage to visual association cortex, and even on the reality of visual agnosia, became widespread.[24] The twentieth-century figure most associated with antilocalization and yet, paradoxically, the teacher of almost all the next generation's leading cortical localizers, was Karl Lashley.

———

Karl Lashley was the first director of the Yerkes Laboratory of Primate Biology in Orange Park, Florida. This was the first U.S. primate center and a joint Harvard-Yale enterprise, Harvard providing the director and Yale providing the laboratory.[25] Until moving to Orange Park, Lashley spent much of his experimental career failing to find evidence for cortical localization of complex behavior in rats.[26] He now set out to resolve the controversy over the localization of visual agnosia by studying the effects of lesions of visual association cortex in monkeys. He tested the monkeys on a rather extensive battery that included tests of sensory status and of visual learning and memory.[27] He had planned to destroy Brodmann's areas 18 and 19 but, as detailed in his classic attack on cytoarchitectonics,[28] he could not identify them reliably. Therefore, he made "no pretense of dealing with a distinct anatomic or functional area," and instead removed "a band of cortex encircling the striate area and extending for an indeterminate distance beyond the lunate sulcus." He coined the term "prestriate region" for this band.[29]

The prestriate lesions in his animals included "not less than 60% of Brodmann's areas 18 and 19" (his estimate), and not much more (my estimate). His "indeterminate" distance included some limited encroachment into posterior parietal and posterior temporal cortex. He found that these lesions[30]:

> did not produce any trace of object agnosia . . . [or] . . . any significant amnesia for . . . color or form . . . interruption of transcortical associative connections is therefore not the cause of visual agnosia [and] comparison of the experimental and clinical evidence indicates that visual agnosia cannot be ascribed to uncomplicated loss of prestriate tissue.

These apparently conclusive antilocalization implications were reversed soon after the arrival in Orange Park in the late 1940s of two graduate students, Josephine Semmes (later Blum) from Yale and Kao Liang Chow from Harvard. They were joined by Karl Pribram, who had trained in neurosurgery with Bucy at Chicago. In a joint study they made lesions much larger than Lashley's, encroaching further into the parietal lobe and much more anteriorly and ventrally into the temporal lobe. These succeeded in producing psychic blindness, that is, severe deficits in visual discrimination learning (as well as some tactile learning deficits that will be discussed later). Since the locus common to their lesions and Klüver and Bucy's was temporal cortex, they surmised that temporal cortex must be crucial for visual learning. Chow then went on to show that, indeed, "lesions of the lateral surface of the temporal lobe and especially the middle temporal gyrus, produced visual deficits," whereas lesions of adjacent areas did not.[31]

In these studies the cortical lesions that led to the visual deficits did not produce any of the other components of the Klüver-Bucy syndrome such as tameness and changes in sexual and eating behaviors. Rather, as Pribram and Bagshaw[32] demonstrated, these components, without the visual difficulties, followed lesions of the amygdala and adjacent cortex. Thus, the original Brown-Schäfer/Klüver-Bucy syndrome was fractionated into visual discrimination difficulties after temporal cortical damage and other, "motivational" symptoms after amygdala damage.

Pribram continued his studies of cortical function in monkeys first in John Fulton's laboratory at Yale and then in a new laboratory established for him at the Institute of Living, a private mental hospital in Connecticut. He was joined by Mortimer Mishkin from McGill University; they further localized the visual components of the Klüver-Bucy syndrome to the middle and inferior temporal gyri.[33] This region became known as inferotemporal cortex or, more recently, inferior temporal (IT) cortex. In the mid-1950s, research on the behavioral effects of IT lesions was also continuing at Orange Park and in Harry Harlow's laboratory at the University of Wisconsin. By the end of the decade the behavioral effects of IT cortex lesions were being studied in laboratories all across the country (e.g., those of Chow at University of Chicago, the Wilsons at Bryn Mawr, Mishkin at NIMH, Donald Meyer at Ohio State University) as well as in England (Weiskrantz at Cambridge University, Ettlinger at Queens Square, London). Much of this effort was directed toward characterizing the visual learning deficit that followed IT lesions. This research has been reviewed by Gross and Dean.[34]

INFERIOR TEMPORAL CORTEX JOINS THE VISUAL SYSTEM

Beyond characterization of the IT deficit, three major advances led to the current period of research on IT cortex. The first was a set of developments that brought IT cortex into anatomical and functional relation with the rest of the visual system. It had long been supposed from degeneration and strychnine neuronography studies that IT cortex might receive visual information from the pulvinar (to which both the superior colliculus and striate cortex project) and from striate cortex over a corticocortical multisynaptic pathway.[35] In 1965 the cortical pathway was established by Kuypers et al. using silver degeneration techniques, as involving two successive synaptic stages in prestriate cortex.[36] The puzzle was that both large lesions of the pulvinar and attempted interruption of the putative corticocortical pathway repeatedly failed to produce the IT deficit on visual learning.[37] One problem was that complete and selective interruption of the corticocortical pathway required complete prestriate lesions, which were technically impossible both because of the extensive infolding in this area and the impossibility of avoiding massive damage to the underlying visual radiations.

In 1966 Mishkin solved this conundrum by disconnecting IT and striate cortex using a crossed-lesion paradigm: the combination of a striate lesion in one hemisphere, an IT lesion in the other hemisphere, and section of the forebrain commissures.[38] The unilateral IT lesion alone had no effect because bilateral lesions are required to produce the IT deficit on visual learning. The unilateral striate lesion alone had no effect because the remaining striate cortex could send visual information to the IT cortex on the same side over the ipsilateral corticocortical route and to the contralateral IT. Lesions of IT alone had no effect on visual learning because each IT cortex still received input from the ipsilateral striate cortex. Similarly, any two of Mishkin's lesion were ineffective. However, the combination of all three lesions resulted in complete interruption of the pathway between striate and IT cortex, and therefore yielded a severe impairment on visual learning.

———

At this time little was known about the visual association cortex or prestriate region lying between (and connecting) striate and IT cortex. As described above, evidence was accumulating from a variety of other species for visuotopically organized cortical areas in addition to striate cortex. Then Cowey demonstrated a visuotopically organized area in the squirrel monkey adjacent to striate cortex, area V2.[39]

A new phase of visual physiology began in the 1970s, when Jon Kaas and John Allman, initially in Woolsey's lab, began their now classic series of studies of extrastriate visual cortex in the owl monkey.[40] They used single-neuron recording rather than evoked potentials and soon freed themselves of the assumption of only two or three visual areas, rapidly finding an amazing multiplicity of visuotopically organized visual areas extending well into the temporal and parietal lobes. Similar extrastriate visual areas were then mapped in the macaque by a number of laboratories, including those of Zeki, Van Essen, Ungerleider, Desimone, and myself, eventually filling much of posterior association cortex with over two dozen visual areas[41] (see figures 5.1 and 5.6).

A second major development in understanding IT cortex was the beginning of its functional subdivision with the discovery by Iwai and Mishkin that it could be divided into a more anterior area corresponding to von Bonin and Bailey's cytoarchitectonic area TE and a more posterior area they called area TEO[42] (see figure 5.1). This latter region has also been called foveal prestriate cortex and posterior IT cortex. Iwai and Mishkin found that TEO lesions had a greater effect on single-pattern discrimination tasks, whereas TE lesions had a greater effect on concurrent discriminations in which the animal is required to learn several discriminations in parallel. They suggested that these results implied greater mnemonic functions for TE and more perceptual functions for TEO.

Alan Cowey and I then set out to characterize further the differences between the effects of these two lesions. We had been together at Cambridge University as Larry Weiskrantz's graduate students. We were joined by two graduate students, Richard Manning, now a research scientist in the U.S.

Medical Corps, and David Bender, now professor of physiology at SUNY Buffalo. We found that lesions of TE and of TEO produced a number of different effects generally supportive of this mnemonic-perceptual distinction. For example, TEO lesions relative to those of TE resulted in greater impairment on single-object and pattern-discrimination learning tasks, less impairment on concurrent visual learning tasks, more disruption by irrelevant stimuli, and less sensitivity to both shock punishment and partial reinforcement.[43]

More recent work suggests that there is a locus especially critical for visual memory in the anterior ventral portion of inferior temporal cortex, that is, in perirhinal cortex, areas 35 and 36. Perirhinal cortex may serve as a major gateway for the pathway between IT cortex and the hippocampus by way of entorhinal cortex. Interactions along some or all of this pathway appear crucial for facilitating long-term storage of visual information in IT cortex.[44]

The third major development was the beginning of studies of the activity of single neurons in IT cortex. For this topic, I now shift into an autobiographical mode.

EARLY STUDIES OF THE ACTIVITY OF SINGLE NEURONS IN IT CORTEX

When I came to MIT as a postdoctoral fellow, I abandoned my previous research area, the frontal lobes, because I despaired of the possibility of doing anything meaningful with them in terms of psychology, anatomy, or physiology. (The successful research program of Patricia Goldman-Rakic[45] demonstrates how wrong this judgment was.) Instead, I turned to the visual functions of the temporal lobe. I started some lesion experiments (mentioned above) and thought it might be valuable to carry out recording studies in parallel. However, I had never done any single-neuron recording and I had no equipment to do so. At this point Hans-Lukas Teuber, head of the Psychology Department, offered to provide the necessary funds and, at least as important, introduced me to George Gerstein, a postdoctoral fellow in Walter Rosenbliths's Communication Biophysics Laboratory in the Research Laboratory of Electronics at MIT.

Gerstein was working on the auditory system of cats and was expert in neuronal recording and analytic techniques.

He and I prepared to record from IT cortex in awake monkeys during the performance of visual discrimination tasks because, as Gerstein often chanted, "the cortex dissolves in anesthesia." We decided to begin by recording surface potentials from IT cortex during visual discrimination learning on the grounds that this would help us to know what to look for with single-unit recording. We found, as Chow[46] had earlier, a few wiggles in the records that mostly indicated, at least to me, the futility of the electrographic approach.[47] In 1964, before we recorded from our first inferotemporal neuron, Gerstein left for the University of Pennsylvania. Since he was now a long-distance collaborator, we decided to radically simplify the planned experiment so that I could carry it out without him. The simplest experiment we could think of was just to ask whether IT neurons responded to visual stimuli and to use anesthetized animals. Since we were in the home of the double dissociation paradigm,[48] we also used auditory stimuli and, in addition, recorded from the superior temporal gyrus, believed to be an auditory analogue of IT cortex.

Soon I was joined by another postdoctoral fellow, Peter Schiller, who was trained as a clinical psychologist and had worked on visual masking. Even for the time, our experiment was certainly simple enough, if not simplistic. For example, the standard stimuli we used were diffuse light, clicks, and tone bursts. Moreover, the eyes were uncorrected and merely covered with a viscous silicone fluid to prevent drying out, and the fovea and other retinal landmarks were not located. The animals were anesthetized and immobilized.

By vigorous averaging of the responses to 100 or more stimulus presentations, we managed to get IT responses to diffuse light in about a quarter of our sample; no IT cells responded to auditory stimuli. We found the opposite pattern in the superior temporal gyrus. For "about 30 units" in IT we tried "moving and stationary circles, edges and bars of light projected on a screen" and found no responses and therefore "an absence of evidence for receptive fields."[49] We interpreted these results as reflecting one or more of the following: (a) "an organization fundamentally different from that found" by Hubel and

Weisel in areas 17, 18, and 19 of the cat; (b) failure to use sufficiently adequate, optimal, or appropriate stimuli; or (c) use of anesthesia.

So we decided to return to our original plan of recording from awake behaving animals and, because of some concurrent experiments on attention and IT lesions, to study unit activity during attention rather than during visual learning. We set up a board in front of the monkeys with little windows or peep holes to which we could apply our eye or present such objects as a finger, a burning Q-Tip, or a bottle brush. Most of the units responded vigorously to such stimuli, and we classified them as attention units because they fired to any stimulus that seemed to draw the animal's attention, or, at least, that would elicit continued staring at the stimulus as reflected on an electrooculogram. These observations were made in several monkeys and with a number of collaborators, such as Peter Schiller, George Gerstein, and Alan Cowey, and were published over a decade later. We interpreted these results as "suggesting that these units either were involved in some attentional mechanism, had foveal receptive fields, or both."[50]

In 1965 I moved to the Psychology Department at Harvard and was joined by Carlos Eduardo Rocha-Miranda from Brazil (who had once worked with Wade Marshall) and by David Bender, from SUNY Buffalo. We were not sure how to test the "some attentional mechanism" hypothesis, so we decided instead to test the foveal receptive field idea by trying once more to plot receptive fields in an immobilized animal. This time we used nitrous oxide and oxygen for anesthesia and we set out to teach ourselves how to use an ophthalmoscope and a retinoscope, find the fovea, use contact lenses, measure expired CO_2, and on and on. (The story of this "learning experience" deserves a stand-up comedy routine. One example: we couldn't find instructions on using a retinoscope that we could understand until we discovered some in a flight surgeon's manual that started: "aim the beam at the center of the patient's chest, then follow the buttons up . . .")

It is interesting to note some other developments during 1965–1969, the period in which we carried out these experiments. In the same building in which I had worked when I came to MIT, Jerry Lettvin was continuing his

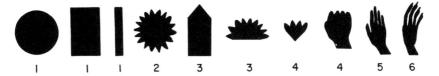

Figure 5.5 Examples of shapes used to stimulate an inferior temporal cortex neuron "apparently having very complex trigger features. The stimuli are arranged from left to right in order of increasing ability to drive the neuron from none (1) or little (2 and 3) to maximum (6). . . . The use of [these] stimuli was begun one day when, having failed to drive a unit with any light stimulus, we waved a hand at the stimulus screen and elicited a very vigorous response from the previously unresponsive neuron. . . . We then spent the next 12 hr testing various paper cutouts in an attempt to find the trigger feature for this unit. When the entire set of stimuli used were ranked according to the strength of the response that they produced, we could not find a simple physical dimension that correlated with this rank order. However, the rank order of adequate stimuli did correlate with similarity (for us) to the shadow of a monkey hand" (Gross et al., 1972).

work on bug detectors in the frog's retina and lecturing (tongue in cheek) on "grandmother cells." Across the river in Harvard Medical School, Hubel and Wiesel had carried out their seminal work on lower- and higher-order complex cells in areas 18 and 19 of the cat. Polish psychologist Jerzy Konorski published his *Integrative Activity of the Brain,* in which he hypothesized a set of gnostic units, neurons that "represented unitary perceptions." He suggested that visual gnostic units were located in inferior temporal cortex, and as likely examples he mentioned units coding faces, hands, and facial expressions. I was well aware of these ideas not only from a stay in his Warsaw laboratory in 1961 but also from reviewing his book.[51]

Given this ambience, it is not surprising that we were prepared to find IT cells that fired selectively to complex stimuli such as hands and faces. The first such cell that we studied in detail was one most responsive to a hand (figure 5.5). When we wrote the first draft of an account of this work for *Science,* we did not have the nerve to include this hand cell until Teuber urged us to do so. What is perhaps more surprising was that for more than a decade there were no published attempts to confirm or deny these and our other early basic results, such as that IT cells have large bilateral fields that include the fovea and are not visuotopically organized. And unlike Panizza, the discoverer of visual cortex in the nineteenth century, we did not publish in obscure journals or from an unknown institution. Perhaps because of the general skepticism, we did not ourselves publish a full account of a face-selective neuron until 1981. Soon thereafter, a flood of papers on such cells appeared, beginning with one by Perrett, Rolls, and Caan from Oxford. Our basic receptive field findings were also first confirmed at that time.[52] To continue our genealogical subtheme, Edmund Rolls was Cowey's student, David Perrett and Woodburn Caan were Rolls's students, and Desimone was my graduate student and Mishkin's post-doctoral student. The laboratories of Rolls in Oxford, Perrett in St. Andrews, and Desimone at the National Institute of Mental Health are today among the most active centers of research on IT cortex.

In the last decade, and therefore beyond our purview, major advances in single-neuron studies of IT cortex have included studies of effects of attention, short-term and long-term memory, specificity for color and faces, functional architecture, and relations with frontal cortex.[53]

A LOST OBSERVATION ON PARIETAL CORTEX

The second set of observations lost in the din of the late nineteenth-century battle between Ferrier and his opponents were made by Ferrier on the effects of lesions of the angular gyrus (posterior parietal cortex) that he thought caused blindness (see figure 1.21). Here is what Ferrier and Yeo had to say about the recovery from this lesion (case 8):

> On the fourth day there were some indications of returning vision. A piece of orange was held before it, whereupon it came forward in a groping manner and tried to lay hold, at first but missed repeatedly . . . On the fifth day . . . *it was evidently able to see its food, but constantly missed laying hold of it* [my italics], putting its hand beyond it or short of it . . . On the sixth day . . . it was able to

pick up grains of rice scattered on the floor, but always with uncertainty as to their exact position . . . Four weeks after the operation . . . the same want of precision was still seen as regards its power of putting its hands on objects it wished to pick up . . . At this date when it was walking on a table it tumbled off, having come too near the edge without seeming to be aware of the fact.

From this description it seems clear that, rather than being blind, this monkey was having problems localizing stimuli and reaching for them. However, since Ferrier had clearly been wrong in localizing the visual center in the parietal lobe, these observations of what he called blindness were usually attributed to some artifact, such as damaging the optic radiations or transiently interfering with occipital function, and then were almost forgotten. In fact Ferrier's opponents, Brown and Schäfer, had made an essentially similar, and even more forgotten, observation, noting that after bilateral posterior parietal lesions, their monkey "would evidently see and run up to [a raisin], but then often fail to find it . . ."[54]

PARIETAL LESIONS IN HUMANS

Thirty years later, at the end of World War I, Sir Gordon Holmes described a group of veterans with disturbances of visual and spatial orientation after bilateral posterior parietal lesions due to penetrating missile wounds. Their symptoms included deficits in reaching and pointing to visual targets, avoiding obstacles, learning and remembering routes, judging distance and size, recognizing spatial relations, fixating a target, and following a moving stimulus. In contrast, their ability to recognize objects and other cognitive functions were essentially normal. Holmes's careful observations established the critical role of posterior parietal cortex in visuospatial functions. His paper was also one of the very few on parietal damage in humans or monkeys that cited Ferrier's early observations on visuospatial deficits after parietal lesions in monkeys.

The next major development was the realization by W. R. Brain, Lord Brain, long-time editor of the journal *Brain,* that unilateral posterior parietal lesions, particularly of the right hemisphere, can produce dramatic neglect of the contralateral side of space. By 1953, the time of Malcolm Critchley's classic monograph *The Parietal Lobes,* it was clear that a variety of complex visual, visuospatial, and visuomotor symptoms occurred after damage to parietal cortex in humans.[55]

PARIETAL CORTEX LESIONS IN THE MONKEY: 20TH CENTURY

The first twentieth-century investigations of posterior parietal cortex function in monkeys were carried out in the 1930s by T. C. Ruch and J. F. Fulton. They found that lesions of this area produced impairments on roughness and weight-discrimination learning. They interpreted these results as indicating that posterior parietal cortex was a somatosensory association area, following the idea that the regions adjacent to each primary sensory area, somatosensory cortex in this case, had the function of developing sensory information into perceptions. Further support for this theory came from studies in Lashley's laboratory in the Yerkes Primate Center, and then in Pribram's laboratory at the Institute of Living. These studies continued to emphasize the role of posterior parietal cortex in tactile learning and indeed, viewed this cortex as playing a role for tactile learning analogous to that of inferior temporal cortex for visual learning. Visuospatial disturbances after parietal lesions were sometimes noticed but usually dismissed as side effects.[56]

The propensity to dismiss the visuospatial effects of posterior parietal lesions as side effects changed with the arrival at Pribram's laboratory of George Ettlinger from the Institute of Neurology, Queens Square, London. He had studied humans with parietal lesions and was aware of Ferrier's earlier observations on the effects of such lesions in monkeys. Ettlinger stressed that the lesions in monkeys produced visual orientation and reaching deficits, and increased sensitivity to stimulus-response separation. He contended that these deficits were the bases of the difficulties in tactile discrimination learning. By the late 1970s several other workers had moved away from the stress on a tactile learning deficit and began to view the deficit as a supramodal spatial one. The beginning of microelectrode studies of parietal cortex tended to strengthen this notion.[57]

THE MICROELECTRODE ARRIVES AT POSTERIOR PARIETAL CORTEX

Single-neuron analysis of posterior parietal cortex began with the work of Juhani Hyvärinen and his colleagues in Helsinki starting in 1970.[58] They found cells that fired:

> . . . when a sensory stimulus which interested the animal was placed in a specific location in space where it became the target of the monkey's gaze or manual reaching, tracking or manipulation . . . Some cells were clearly related to eye movements whereas others appeared to discharge in response to visual sensory stimuli.

They interpreted their results as indicating that posterior parietal cortex was involved in the visuospatial guidance of movement, thereby providing an explanation for the visuospatial deficit after parietal lesions. However, their procedures were somewhat naturalistic: eye and arm movements and position were not measured or controlled, and stimulus presentation was often informal.

Soon after, Vernon Mountcastle and his colleagues at Johns Hopkins explored similar phenomena, and did so under greater experimental control. They found cells specifically related to projection of the arm, to hand manipulation, to visual tracking, and to visual fixation, as well as cells with more complex properties.[59–61] At least in their early papers, they claimed that very few if any of their cells were "directly activated" by visual stimuli. Rather, they described their parietal cells as[62, 63]:

> . . . function[ing] in a command fashion, directing visual attention to and exploration of the immediately surrounding extrapersonal space.

and

> . . . execut[ing] a matching function between the neural signals of
> the nature of objects and the internal drive states of the organism,
> and contain[ing] a neural apparatus for the direction of visual
> attention to objects of interest and for shifting the focus of attention
> from one to another.

Michael Goldberg and David Robinson at the National Institutes of
Health then demonstrated that Mountcastle and his colleagues were quite
wrong: many posterior parietal neurons did in fact respond to visual stimuli and
did so in the absence of movement, thereby unambiguously falsifying the
"motor command" hypothesis. They did find that the visual responses could
often be enhanced by the animal's attention, but this did not necessarily involve
any eye movement at all. Thus Goldberg and Robinson returned posterior
parietal cortex to the visual system where Ferrier first placed it.[64]
    The next decade saw several further significant developments on these
issues. As they are outside of our time frame, I mention only two of them.
First, Andersen and his colleagues showed that the visual responses of posterior
parietal neurons can be modulated by eye position, and therefore an ensemble
of such cells carries information about visual targets in spatial coordinates.
Second, it became clear that there are a number of different visual areas in the
posterior parietal cortex that appear to play different roles in a variety of visual
and visuospatial functions, such as the analysis of stimulus movement, the
coding of space, and the visual control and monitoring of eye and hand
movement.[65]

Coda: Two Cortical Visual Systems

By the early 1980s, the end of the period covered by this book, more than a
dozen cortical visual areas had been described, extending visual cortex from the
occipital lobe well into the temporal and parietal lobes. In 1982, Leslie Unger-

leider and Mortimer Mishkin proposed a powerful and highly influential theory that brought considerable order to this plethora. They proposed that the various extrastriate visual areas could be grouped into two processing "streams" or "systems." The first was a dorsal pathway from striate cortex, through a set of dorsal prestriate areas to posterior parietal cortex, forming a system for spatial vision. The second was a ventral pathway from striate cortex through a set of ventral prestriate area to inferior temporal cortex, forming a system for object vision. Their theory had two major roots. The first was the confirmation and extension in Mishkin's laboratory of the two lost nineteenth-century observations, that inferior temporal lesions produce a psychic blindness for recognizing objects and that posterior parietal lesions produce a deficit in spatial vision. The second root was the proposal made in the late 1960s by Gerald Schneider (my first graduate student) and Colwyn Trevarthen that visual function could be divided into *what?* (or identity) functions and *where?* (or localization) functions, and that these two functions were subserved by different brain structures.[66]

Ungerleider and Mishkin's "two visual systems" has sometimes been simplified to the point of caricature by others, and therefore several caveats should be kept in mind, most of which were explicit or implicit in their original or subsequent formulations.[67] First, both the dorsal and ventral systems are interconnected along their entire course and must continually interact; that is, they are "bound" to each other just as objects are to their locations. Second, each is undoubtedly subdivided. For example, evidence exists for two streams within the dorsal system, one specialized for space and proceeding to posterior parietal cortex and one specialized for analysis of stimulus movement and proceeding to the superior temporal polysensory (STP) area in the anterior portion of the upper bank of the superior temporal sulcus.[68] Third, even within a stream or substream, processing is probably parallel as well as serial. Thus, the analysis of form and color proceeds somewhat separately in the early stages of the ventral system,[69] and in the later stages there are several routes to anterior IT cortex.[70] See figure 5.6.

A fourth point to remember about the two cortical visual systems schema is that the dorsal and ventral streams do not end in parietal and temporal cortex.

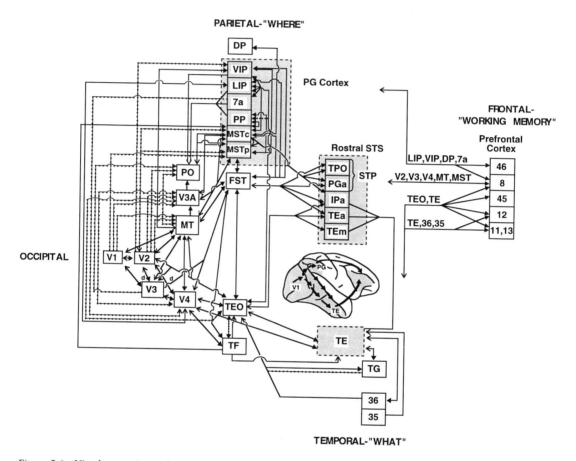

Figure 5.6 Visual processing pathways in monkeys. Solid lines indicate connections from both central and peripheral visual field representations; dotted lines indicate connections from only peripheral representations. Shaded regions on the lateral view of the brain show the extent of cortex represented in the diagram. The locations of many of these areas and their abbreviations are shown in figure 5.1 (updated after Ungerleider, 1995, courtesy, L. Ungerleider).

Rather, they continue into the frontal lobe, the dorsal stream to the dorsolateral and dorsomedial region, and the ventral stream to the ventrolateral and orbital region.[71] Furthermore, lesion and neuronal recording studies indicate that these dorsal and ventral frontal areas retain their specialization for spatial and object vision, respectively.[72] Fifth, the dorsal and ventral systems even segregate their limbic connections, IT projecting primarily to the perirhinal area (areas 35/36) which then projects to the anterior 2/3 of entorhinal cortex and posterior parietal, projecting primarily to the parahippocampal cortex (area TF) which projects to the posterior 2/3 of entorhinal cortex.[73] At least some of this segregation is maintained in the hippocampus itself.[74]

Sixth, and finally, beware the reification of categories: the dorsal stream is crucial for visuomotor function, as well as spatial vision, as Ferrier noticed and Melvin Goodale and David Milner[75] recently stressed; structure from motion requires the ventral system[76] and MT can use wavelength information.[77,78]

NOTES

1. Lashley, 1950.

2. Morgan and Stellar, 1950.

3. Kreig, 1975.

4. Teuber, 1955.

5. Gross, 1987a.

6. Broca, 1861; Young, 1970b.

7. Fritsch and Hitzig, 1870.

8. Flechsig, 1886.

9. Boring, 1950.

10. Hume, 1739; Titchener, 1910.

11. Bolton, 1900; Campbell, 1905.

12. Elliot-Smith, 1907.

13. Brodmann, 1909; von Economo, 1929.

14. James, 1890.

15. Talbot and Marshall, 1941.

16. Hubel and Wiesel, 1965.

17. Brown and Schäfer, 1888.

18. E.g., Schäfer, 1988a, b, 1900.

19. Klüver, 1933.

20. Klüver, 1926, 1928.

21. Klüver and Bucy, 1938, 1939.

22. Klüver, 1948.

23. Goltz, 1888; Loeb, 1900. Loeb started his career by studying the effects of brain lesions in dogs under Goltz. Inspired by work on plant tropism, Loeb (1900) then developed his theory of animal tropisms, which tried to explain at least simple behaviors in terms of common physical and chemical forces acting on the organism. He came to America in 1891, where his mechanistic theories of behavior had considerable impact, memorably on W. B. Crozier and the young men around him at Harvard, particularly B. F. Skinner (Pauly, 1990). Loeb was the model for Gottlieb in Sinclair Lewis's (1925) novel about medical research, *Arrowsmith*. Crozier was part of the model for Burris in Skinner's utopian novel *Walden Two* (1948) Skinner himself being the other part (Skinner, 1984).

24. E.g., Goldstein, 1939; Bender and Feldman, 1972.

25. Lashley had been appointed to Harvard in 1935 as a result of its president's demand for "the best psychologist in the world" (Boring et al., 1952). A few years later he seems to have had enough of the Boston brahmins and clinical psychologists in the Department of Psychology, and was delighted to confine his teaching in Cambridge to two weeks a year and spend the rest of his time in Orange Park, Florida.

26. Lashley, 1933, 1950.

27. Lashley, 1948.

28. Lashley and Clark, 1946.

29. Lashley, 1948.

30. Lashley, 1948.

31. Blum et al., 1950; Chow, 1951.

32. Pribram and Bagshaw, 1953.

33. Mishkin and Pribram, 1954; Mishkin, 1954.

34. Gross, 1973, 1994b; Dean, 1976.

35. Chow and Hutt, 1953.

36. Kuypers et al., 1965.

37. E.g., Chow, 1961.

38. Mishkin, 1966.

39. Cowey, 1964.

40. Allman and Kaas, 1971; Kaas, 1997.

41. For a discussion of the converging criteria for extrastriate visual areas, see Gross et al. (1993). For reviews of the properties and connections of these areas, see Felleman and Van Essen (1991), and Desimone and Ungerleider (1989).

42. Mishkin, 1966; von Bonin and Bailey, 1947; Iwai and Mishkin, 1968.

43. See references in Gross, 1973.

44. E.g., Meunier et al., 1993; Suzuki and Amaral, 1994.

45. Goldman-Rakic, 1987.

46. Chow, 1961.

47. Gerstein et al., 1969.

48. Teuber, 1955.

49. Gross et al., 1967.

50. Gross et al., 1979.

51. Lettvin et al., 1959; Lettvin, 1995; Hubel and Wiesel, 1965; Konorski, 1967; Gross, 1992; Barlow, 1995; Gross, 1968.

52. Gross et al., 1969, 1972; Bruce et al., 1981; Perrett et al., 1982; Desimone, 1991; Desimone and Gross, 1979, Richmond and Wurtz, 1982.

53. E.g., Miyashita, 1993; Tanaka, 1996; Gross et al., 1993; Desimone et al., 1995.

54. Ferrier and Yeo, 1884; Brown and Schäfer, 1888.

55. Holmes, 1918b; Brain, 1941; Critchley, 1953.

56. E.g., Ruch et al., 1938; Blum et al., 1950; Blum, 1951; Wilson, 1957; Wilson et al., 1960.

57. Bates and Ettlinger, 1960; Ettlinger and Kahlsbeck, 1962; Ettlinger et al., 1966; Semmes, 1965; Milner et al., 1977.

58. Hyvärinen and Poranen, 1974; reviewed in Hyvärinen, 1982.

59. Mountcastle, 1976.

60. Mountcastle et al., 1975.

61. Lynch et al., 1977.

62. Mountcastle et al., 1975.

63. Lynch et al., 1977.

64. Goldberg and Robinson, 1977, 1980; Robinson et al., 1978; Bushnell et al., 1981.

65. First, Andersen et al., 1985; second, Colby and Duhamel, 1991; Gross and Graziano, 1994; Duhamel et al., 1992.

66. Ungerleider and Mishkin, 1982; Schneider, 1967; Trevarthen, 1968.

67. Macko et al. 1982, Desimone and Ungerleider, 1989.

68. Bruce et al., 1981; Graziano and Gross, 1995.

69. Livingstone and Hubel, 1988.

70. E.g., Martin-Elkins and Horel, 1992.

71. Macko et al., 1982; Barbas, 1988; Webster et al., 1994; Rodman, 1994.

72. E.g., Gross and Weiskrantz, 1964; Wilson et al., 1993; Goldman-Rakic, 1987; Mishkin and Manning, 1978.

73. Suzuki and Amaral, 1994.

74. Witter and Amaral, 1991.

75. Goodale and Milner, 1992.

76. Britten et al., 1992.

77. Dobkins and Albright, 1994.

78. After this book went to press, Nahm (1997) published a detailed account of Kluver's discovery of the temporal lobe syndrome in which he suggests a perceived similarity in "lip smacking" after mescaline and in temporal lobe epilepsy contributed to the discovery.

REFERENCES

[Anonymous, 1844]. Review of Swedenborg E., *The Animal Kingdom. Athenaeum,* Jan. 20, 1844. p. 61.

[Anonymous, 1863]. Review of T. H. Huxley, *Evidence as to man's place in nature. Anthropol. Rev.* 1:107–117.

Ackerman, J. S., 1978. Leonardo's eye. *J. Warburg Courtauld Inst.* 41:108–146.

Acton, A., 1938. Preface to Swedenborg E., *Three Transactions on the Cerebrum.* A. Acton, trans. Swedenborg Scientific Association, Philadelphia.

Adrian, E. D., 1928. *The Basis of Sensation.* Christophers, London.

Adrian, E. D., 1947. *The Physical Background of Perception.* Clarendon Press, Oxford.

Adrian, E. D., and Matthews, B., 1927. The action of light on the eye. Part 1. The discharge of impulses in the optic nerve and its relation to the electric changes in the retina. *J. Physiol.* 97:378–414.

Akert, K., and Hammond, M. P., 1962. Emanuel Swedenborg (1688–1772) and his contribution to neurology. *Med. Hist.* 2:255–266.

Allman, J. M., and Kaas, J. H., 1971. A representation of the visual field in the caudal third of the middle temporal gyrus of the owl monkey (*Aotus trivirgatus*). *Brain Res.* 31:85–101.

Andersen, R. A., Essick, G. K., and Siegel, R. M., 1985. Encoding of spatial location by posterior parietal neurons. *Science* 230:456–458.

Avicenna [Ibn Sina], 1930 [11th C.]. *The Canon of Medicine*. O. C. Gruner, trans. Luzac, London.

Barbas, H., 1988. Anatomic organization of basoventral and mediodorsal visual recipient prefrontal regions in the rhesus monkey. *J. Comp. Neurol.* 276:313–342.

Barlow, H. B., 1953. Summation and inhibition in the frog's retina. *J. Physiol.* 119:69–88.

Barlow, H. B., 1995. The neuron doctrine in perception. In: *The Cognitive Neurosciences*. M. S. Gazzaniga, ed. MIT Press, Cambridge.

Bartholin, T., 1656. *Anatomia reformata*. Quotation translated in: The rise of the "enteroid process" in the 19th century: some landmarks in cerebral nomenclature. F. Schiller (1965). *Bull. Hist. Med.* 41:515–538.

Bartley, S. H., 1934. Relation of intensity and duration of brief retinal stimulation by light to the electrical response of the optic cortex of the rabbit. *Am. J. Physiol.* 108:397–408.

Barton, R., 1990, An influential set of chaps: The X Club and Royal Society politics 1864–85. *Br. J. Hist. Sci.* 23:53–81.

Bates, J. A. V., and Ettlinger, G., 1960. Posterior biparietal ablations in the monkey. *Arch. Neurol.* 3:177–192.

Beare, J. I., 1906. *Greek Theories of Elementary Cognition from Alcmaeon to Aristotle*. Clarendon Press, Oxford.

Beck, A., 1890. Die Bestimmung der Localisation der Gehirn und Rückenmarkfunctionen vermittelst der elektrischen Erscheinungen. *Cent. Physiol.* 4:473–476.

———

Beck, A., 1973. The Determination of Localizations in the Brain and Spinal Cord with the Aid of Electrical Phenomena. M. A. B. Brazier, trans. *Acta Neurobiol. Exp. Suppl.* 3:7–56.

Bell, C., 1811. *Idea of a New Anatomy of the Brain.* Warren and Son, Winchester.

Bell, C., 1812. Idea of a new anatomy of the brain. *Balt. Med. Phil. Lyceum* 1:303–318.

Bender, M. B., and Feldman, M., 1972. The so-called "visual agnosia." *Brain* 95:173–186.

Bennett, J. H., 1837. *On the Physiology and Pathology of the Brain: Being an Attempt to Ascertain what Portions of the Brain Are more Immediately Connected with Motion, Sensation, and Intelligence.* Carfrae, Edinburgh.

Bibby, C., 1959. *T. H. Huxley, Scientist, Humanist and Educator.* Watts, London.

[Blake, C., 1863]. Review of *Evidence as to Man's Place in Nature. Edinb. Rev.* 117:541–569.

Blinderman, C. S., 1957. The Oxford debate and after. *Notes and Queries,* March 1957, 126–128.

Blinderman, C. S., 1971. The great bone case. *Perspect. Biol. Med.* 14:370–393.

Blum, J. S., 1951. Cortical organization in somesthesis: Effects of lesions in posterior associative cortex on somatosensory function in *Macaca mulatta. Comp. Psychol. Monogr.* 20:219–249.

Blum, J. S., Chow, K. L., and Pribram, K. H., 1950. A behavioral analysis of the organization of the parieto-temporo-preoccipital cortex. *J. Comp. Neurol.* 93:53–100.

Boakes, R. A., 1984. *From Darwin to Behaviorism: Psychology and the Minds of Animals.* Cambridge University Press, Cambridge.

Bolton, J. S., 1900. The exact histological localization of the visual area of the human cerebral cortex. *Phil. Trans. R. Soc. Lond.* 193:165–222.

Boring, E. G., 1942. *Sensation and Perception in the History of Experimental Psychology.* Appleton-Century-Crofts, New York.

Boring, E. G., 1950. *A History of Experimental Psychology.* Appleton-Century-Crofts, New York.

Boring, E. G., Langfeld, H. S., and Yerkes, R. M., 1952. *A History of Psychology in Autobiography,* Vol. 4. Clark University Press, Worcester, MA.

Brain, W. R., 1941. Visual disorientation with special reference to lesions of the right cerebral hemisphere. *Brain* 64:244–272.

Brazier, M. A. B., 1988. *A History of Neurophysiology in the Nineteenth Century.* Raven Press, New York.

Breasted, J. H., 1930. *The Edwin Smith Surgical Papyrus.* University of Chicago Press, Chicago.

Britten, K. H., Newsome, W. T., and Saunders, R. C., 1992. Effects of inferotemporal cortex lesions on form-from-motion discrimination in monkeys. *Exp. Brain Res.* 88:292–302.

Broca, P., 1861. Remarks on the seat of the faculty of articulate language, followed by an observation of aphemia. In: *Some Papers on the Cerebral Cortex.* G. Von Bonin (1960), trans. Charles C. Thomas, Springfield, IL.

Brodmann, K., 1909. *Vergleichende Lokalisationslehre der Grosshirnrinde in ihren Prinzipien dargestellt auf Grund des Zellenbaues.* Barth, Leipzig.

Brown, J., 1995. *Charles Darwin: Voyaging.* Knopf, New York.

Brown, S., and Schäfer, E. A., 1888. An investigation into the functions of the occipital and temporal lobes of the monkey's brain. *Phil. Trans. R. Soc. Lond.* 179:303–327.

Bruce, C., Desimone, R., and Gross, C. G., 1981. Visual properties of neurons in a polysensory area in superior temporal sulcus of the macaque. *J. Neurophysiol.* 46:369–384.

Burkhardt, F. H., and Smith, S. 1985–. *The Correspondence of Charles Darwin*. Cambridge University Press, Cambridge.

Burton, R. F., trans., 1885. *The Book of the Thousand Nights and a Night,* Vol. 5. Burton Club, London.

Bush, G., 1847. *Mesmer and Swedenborg or the Relation of the Developments of Mesmerism to the Doctrines of Disclosures of Swedenborg.* John Allen, New York.

Bushnell, M. C., Goldberg, M. E., and Robinson, D. L., 1981. Behavioral enhancement of visual responses in monkey cerebral cortex, I. Modulation in posterior parietal cortex related to selective visual attention. *J. Neurophysiol.* 46:755–772.

Calder, R., 1970. *Leonardo and the Age of the Eye*. Simon and Schuster, New York.

Campbell, A. W., 1905. *Histological Studies on the Localization of Cerebral Function*. Cambridge University Press, Cambridge.

Canfora, L., 1990. *The Vanished Library.* M. Ryle, trans. University of California Press, Berkeley.

Carpenter, M. B., and Sutin, J. 1983. *Human Neuroanatomy,* 8th ed. Williams & Wilkins, Baltimore.

Carpenter, W. B., 1845. *Principles of Human Physiology.* Lea & Blanchard, Philadelphia.

Caton, R., 1875. The electric currents of the brain. *Br. Med. J.* 2:278.

Chang, J., 1977. *The Tao of Love and Sex.* Wildwood, Aldershot, UK.

Chambers, R., 1844. *Vestiges of the Natural History of Creation.* Reprinted 1969. Leicester University Press, Leicester.

Chow, K-L., 1951. Effects of partial extirpations of the posterior association cortex on visually mediated behavior. *Comp. Psychol. Monogr.* 20:187–217.

———

Chow, K-L., 1961. Anatomical and electrographical analysis of temporal neocortex in relation to visual discrimination learning in monkeys. In: *Brain Mechanisms and Learning.* J. Delafresnay, ed. Blackwell, Oxford.

Chow, K-L. and Hutt, P., 1953. The "association Cortex" of *Macaca mulatta:* A review of recent contributions to its anatomy and functions. *Brain* 76:625–677.

Church, W. S., 1861. On the myology of the orangutan. *Nat. Hist. Rev.* 1:510–515.

Clark, K. A., 1935. *Catalogue of the Drawings of Leonardo da Vinci at Windsor Castle.* Cambridge University Press, Cambridge.

Clark, K. A., 1939. *Leonardo da Vinci, an Account of His Development as an Artist.* Cambridge University Press, Cambridge.

Clarke, E., 1962. The early history of cerebral ventricles. *Trans. Stud. Coll. Phys. Phila.* 30:85–89.

Clarke, E., 1963. Aristotelian concepts of the form and functions of the brain. *Bull. Hist. Med.* 37:1–14.

Clarke, E., and Bearn, J. G., 1968. The brain "glands" of Malpighi elucidated by practical history. *J. Hist. Med. Allied Sci.* 23:309–330.

Clarke, E., and Dewhurst, K. E., 1996. *An Illustrated History of Brain Function.* Norman, San Francisco.

Clarke, E., and Jacyna, L. S., 1987. *Nineteenth-century Origins of Neuroscientific Concepts.* University of California Press, Berkeley.

Clarke, E., and O'Malley, C. D., 1996. *The Human Brain and Spinal Cord, a Histological Study Illustrated by Writings from Antiquity to the Twentieth Century.* Norman, San Francisco.

Clarke, E., and Stannard, J., 1963. Aristotle on the anatomy of the brain. *J. Hist. Med.* 18:130–148.

———

Clayton, M., 1992. *Leonardo da Vinci: The Anatomy of Man*. Little, Brown, Boston.

Colby, C. L., and Duhamel, J. R., 1991. Heterogeneity of extrastriate visual areas and multiple parietal areas in the macaque monkey. *Neuropsychologia* 29:517–537.

Coleman, W., 1971. *Biology in the Nineteenth Century: Problems of Form, Function and Transformation*. Wiley, New York.

Combe, G., 1852. *Lectures on Phrenology*. Fowlers and Wells, New York.

Cooter, R. S., 1985. *The Cultural Meaning of Popular Science: Phrenology and the Organization of Consent in Nineteenth-century Britain*. Cambridge University Press, Cambridge.

Corner, G. W., 1927. *Anatomical Texts of the Earlier Middle Ages: A Study in the Transmission of Culture*. Carnegie Institute of Washington, Washington, DC.

Cowey, A., 1964. Projection of the retina onto striate and prestriate cortex in the squirrel monkey, *Saimiri sciureus*. *J. Neurophysiol.* 27:366–393.

Cranefield, P. F., 1974. *The Way In and the Way Out: Francois Magendie, Charles Bell and the Roots of the Spinal Nerves*. Futura, Mount Kisco, NY.

Critchley, M., 1953. *The Parietal Lobes*. Arnold, London.

Daniel, P. M., and Whitteridge, D., 1961. The representation of the visual field on the cerebral cortex in monkeys. *J. Physiol.* 159:203–221.

Darwin, C., 1861. *The Origin of Species*. Murray, London.

Darwin, C., 1871. *The Descent of Man and Selection in Relation to Sex*. Murray, London.

Darwin, C., 1909. *The Origin of Species,* with additions and corrections from the 6th English ed. Appleton-Century-Crofts, New York.

Darwin, F., 1887. *The Life and Letters of Charles Darwin*. Murray, London.

Darwin, F., 1903. *More Letters of Charles Darwin*. Appleton-Century-Crofts, New York.

Dean, P., 1976. Effects of inferotemporal lesions on the behavior of monkeys. *Psychol. Bull.* 83:41–71.

Descartes, R., 1972 [1662]. *Treatise on Man*. T. S. Hall, trans. Harvard University Press, Cambridge.

Desimone, R., 1991. Face-selective cells in the temporal cortex of monkeys. *J. Cognit. Neurosci.* 3:1–8.

Desimone, R., and Gross, C. G., 1979. Visual areas in the temporal cortex of the macaque. *Brain Res.* 78:363–380.

Desimone, R., Miller, E. K., Chelazzi, L., and Lueschow, A., 1995. Multiple memory systems in the visual cortex. In: *The Cognitive Neurosciences*. M. Gazzaniga, ed. MIT Press, Cambridge.

Desimone, R., and Ungerleider, L. G., 1989. Neural mechanisms of visual processing in monkeys. In: *Handbook of Neurophysiology*, Vol. 2. F. Boller and J. Grafman, eds. Elsevier Science Publishers, Essex.

Desmond, A., 1984. *Archetypes and Ancestors*. University of Chicago Press, Chicago.

Desmond, A., 1989. Lamarckism and democracy: Corporations, corruption, and comparative anatomy in the 1830s. In: *History, Humanity, and Evolution: Essays in Honor of John C. Greene*. J. R. Moore, ed. Cambridge University Press, Cambridge.

Desmond, A., 1992. *The Politics of Evolution: Morphology, Medicine, and Reform in Radical London*. University of Chicago Press, Chicago.

Desmond, A., 1994. *Huxley: The Devil's Disciple*. Michael Joseph, London.

Desmond, A., and Moore, J. R., 1992. *Darwin: The Life of a Tortured Evolutionist*. Warner, New York.

Devereux, D. and Pellegrin, P., eds., 1990. *Biologie, Logique et Metaphysique chez Aristotle.* Editions CNRS, Paris.

De Viessens, R., 1685. *Neurographia Universalis.* Certe, Lyons.

Dewhurst, K. E., 1982. Thomas Willis and the foundations of British neurology. In: *Historical Aspects of the Neurosciences.* F. Rose and W. Bynum, eds. Raven Press, New York.

Diamond, J., 1992. *The Third Chimpanzee.* Harper Collins, New York.

Diderot, D., and D'Alembert, J., 1751. *Encyclopedia ou Dictionairre Raisonne des Sciences, des Artes, et des Metiers.* Pellet, Geneva.

DiGregorio, M. A., 1984. *T. H. Huxley's Place in Natural Science.* Yale University Press, New Haven, CT.

Dingle, H., 1958. The scientific work of Emanuel Swedenborg. *Endeavour* 17:127–132.

Disraeli, B., 1847. *Tancred, or the New Crusade.* Colburn, London.

Dobkins, K., and Albright, T., 1994. What happens if it changes color when it moves? The nature of chromatic input to macaque visual area MT. *J. Neurosci.* 14:4854–4870.

Dobson, J. F., 1926–1927. Erasistratus. *Proc. R. Soc. Med.* 20:825–832.

Dow, R. S., 1940. Thomas Willis (1621–1675) as a comparative neurologist. *Ann. Med. Hist.* 2:181–194.

Duhamel, J. R, Colby, C. L., and Goldberg, M. E., 1992. The updating of the representation of visual space in parietal cortex by intended eye movements. *Science* 255:90–92.

Eastwood, B., 1985. Al-Hazen, Leonardo and late-medieval speculation on the inversion of images in the eye. *Ann. Sci.* 43:413–446.

Edelstein, L., 1967a. The history of anatomy in antiquity. In: *Ancient Medicine, Selected Papers of Ludwig Edelstein*. O. Temkin and C. Temkin, eds. Johns Hopkins University Press, Baltimore.

Edelstein, L., 1967b. The Hippocratic Oath: Text, translations and interpretation. In *Ancient Medicine, Selected Papers of Ludwig Edelstein*. O. Temkin and C. Temkin, eds. Johns Hopkins University Press, Baltimore.

[Egerton, P.], 1861. Monkeyana. *Punch,* May 18, 1861.

Eiseley, L., 1961. *Darwin's Century.* Doubleday, Garden City, NY.

Ellegard, A., 1958. *Darwin and the General Reader: The Reception of Darwin's Theory of Evolution in the British Periodical Press, 1859–1872.* Göteborgs Universitets Arsskrift, Göteborgs.

Elliot Smith, G., 1907. New studies on the folding of the visual cortex and the significance of the occipital sulci in the human brain. *J. Anat.* 41: 198–207.

Ettlinger, G., and Kahlsbeck, J. E., 1962. Changes in tactual discrimination and in visual reaching after successive and simultaneous bilateral posterior parietal ablations in the monkey, *J. Neurol. Neurosurg. Psychiatry* 25:256–268.

Ettlinger, G., Morton, H. B., and Moffett, E., 1966. Tactile discrimination performance in the monkey. The effect of bilateral posterior parietal and lateral frontal ablations, and of callosal section. *Cortex* 2:5–29.

Farrington, B., 1944. Greek science. 1 *Thales to Aristotle.* Penguin, Harmondsworth.

Farrington, B., 1949. Greek science. 2 *Theopharastus to Galen.* Penguin, Harmondsworth.

Felleman, D. J., and Van Essen, D. C., 1991. Distributed hierarchical processing in primate cerebral cortex. *Cereb. Cortex* 1:1–48.

Ferrier, D., 1873. Experimental researches in cerebral physiology and pathology. *West Riding Lunatic Asylum Med. Rep.* 3:30–96

Ferrier, D., 1875a. On the brain of monkeys. *Proc. R. Soc. Lond.* 23:409–432.

Ferrier, D., 1875b. Experiments on the brain of monkeys. *Phil. Trans. R. Soc. Lond.* 165:433–488.

Ferrier, D., 1876. *Functions of the Brain,* 1st ed. Smith and Elder, London.

Ferrier, D., 1878. *The Localisation of Cerebral Disease.* Smith and Elder, London.

Ferrier, D., 1886. *Functions of the Brain,* 2nd ed. Smith and Elder, London.

Ferrier, D., 1888. Schäfer on the temporal and occipital lobes. *Brain* 11:7–30.

Ferrier, D., and Yeo, G. F., 1884. A record of the experiments on the effects of lesions of different regions of the cerebral hemispheres. *Phil. Trans. R. Soc. Lond.* 175:479–564.

Flechsig, P., 1886. *Gehirn und Steele.* Veit, Leipzig.

Fletcher, J., 1835. *Rudiments of Physiology.* Carfrae, Edinburgh.

Flower, W. H., 1862. On the posterior lobes of the cerebrum of the *Quadrumana. Phil. Trans. R. Soc. Lond.* 152:185–201.

Foster, M., 1901. *Lectures on the History of Physiology During the 16th, 17th and 18th Centuries.* Cambridge University Press, Cambridge.

Fraser, P., 1972. *Ptolemaic Egypt.* Oxford University Press, Oxford.

Freeman, K., 1954. *The Pre-Socratic Philosophers.* Blackwell, Oxford.

Freud, S., 1953, [1891]. *On Aphasia: A Critical Study.* International University Press, New York.

Fritsch, G. T, and Hitzig, E., 1870. On the electrical excitability of the cerebrum. In: *Some Papers on the Cerebral Cortex.* G. von Bonin (1960), trans. Charles C Thomas, Springfield, IL.

Fulton, J. F., 1937. A note on Franesco Gennari and the early history of cytoarchitectonic studies of the cerebral cortex *Bull. Inst. Hist. Med.* 5:895–913.

Galen, 1541. *Omnia Opera.* Giunta, Venice.

Galen, 1956 [2nd C.]. *On Anatomical Procedures, the Surviving Books.* W. L. H. Duckworth, trans. Oxford University Press, Oxford.

Galen, 1962 [2nd C.]. *On Anatomical Procedures, the Later Books.* C. Singer, trans. Cambridge University Press, Cambridge.

Galen, 1968 [2nd C.]. *On the Usefullness of the Parts of the Body.* M. May, trans. Cornell University Press, Ithaca, NY.

Galen, 1978–1984 [2nd C.]. *On the Doctrines of Hippocrates and Plato.* P. DeLacy, trans. Akademie-Verkag, Berlin.

Gall, F. J., and Spurzheim, J. C., 1810. *Anatomie et Physiologie du Systeme Nerveux.* Schoell, Paris.

Gall, F. J., and Spurzheim, J. C., 1835. *On the Function of the Brain and Each of Its Parts: With Observations on the Possibility of Determining the Instincts, Propensities and Talents, or the Moral and Intellectual Dispositions of Men and Animals, by the Configuration of the Brain and Head.* W. Lewis, Jr., trans. Marsh, Capen, and Lyon, Boston.

Gattass, R., Gross, C. G., and Sandell, J. H., 1981. Visual topography of V2 in the macaque. *J. Comp. Neurol.* 201:519–539.

Gennari, F., 1782. *De Peculiari Structura Cerebri Nonnullisque Eius Morbis.* Ex. Regio Typogratheo, Parma.

Gerstein, G. L., Gross, C. G., and Weinstein, M., 1969. Inferotemporal evoked potentials during visual discrimination performance by monkeys. *J. Comp. Physiol. Psychol.* 65:526–528.

Glickstein, M., and Rizzolatti, G., 1984. Francesco Gennari and the structure of the cerebral cortex. *Trends Neurosci.* 7:464–467.

Glickstein, M., and Whitteridge, D., 1987. Tatsuji Inouye and the mapping of the visual fields on the human cerebral cortex. *Trends Neurosci.* 10:350–353.

Goldberg, M. E., and Robinson, D. L., 1977. Visual responses of neurons in monkey inferior parietal lobule: The physiologic substrate of attention and neglect, *Neurology* 27:350.

Goldberg, M. E., and Robinson, D. L., 1980. The significance of enhanced visual responses in posterior parietal cortex. *Behav. Brain Sci.* 3:503–505.

Goldman-Rakic, P. S., 1987. Circuitry of primate prefrontal cortex and regulation of behavior by representational memory. In: *Handbook of Physiology: The Nervous System,* Vol. 5. V. B. Mountcastle, ed. American Physiological Society, Bethesda.

Goldstein, K., 1939. *The Organism.* American Book Co., New York.

Goltz, F., 1888. On the functions of the hemispheres. In: *Some Papers on the Cerebral Cortex.* G. von Bonin (1960), trans. Charles C Thomas, Springfield, IL.

Goodale, M. A., and Milner, A. D., 1992. Separate visual pathways for perception and action. *Trends Neurosci.* 15:20–25.

Gotthelf, A., and Lennox, J. G., eds., 1987. *Philosophical Issues in Aristotle's Biology.* Cambridge University Press, Cambridge.

Gould, S. J., 1981. *The Mismeasure of Man.* Norton, New York.

Gould, S. J., 1982. The Hottentot Venus. *Nat. His.* 91(10):20–27.

Gould, S. J., 1986. Knight takes Bishop. *Nat. Hist.* 95(5):18–33.

Gratiolet, P., 1854. Note sur les expansions des racines cérébrales du nerf optique et sur leur terminaison dans une région determinée de l'écorce des hemisphères. *Compt. Rend. Acad. Sci.* 39:274–278.

Graziano, M. S. A., and Gross, C. G., 1995. From eye to hand. In: *Scale in Conscious Experience: Is the Brain too Important to Be Left to Specialists to Study?* Lawrence Erlbaum Assoc., Mahwah, NJ.

Grene, M., 1963. *A Portrait of Aristotle.* Faber and Faber, London.

Gross, C. G., 1968. Review of J. Konorski, *Integrative Activity of the Brain* (1967). *Science* 160:652–653.

Gross, C. G., 1973. Visual functions of inferotemporal cortex. In: *Handbook of Sensory Physiology,* Vol. VII/3B. H. Autrum, R. Jung, W. Lowenstein, D. McKay, and H.-L. Teuber, eds. Springer-Verlag, Berlin.

Gross, C. G., 1981. Ibn-al-Haytham on eye and brain, vision and perception. *Bull. Islamic Med.* 1:309–312.

Gross, C. G., 1987a. Phrenology. In: *Encyclopedia of Neuroscience.* G. Adelman, ed. Birkhauser, Boston.

Gross, C. G., 1987b. Early history of neuroscience. In: *Encyclopedia of Neuroscience.* G. Adelman, ed. Birkhauser, Boston.

Gross, C. G., 1992. Representation of visual stimuli in inferior temporal cortex. *Phil. Trans. R. Soc. Lond.* 335:3–10.

Gross, C. G., 1993a. Hippocampus minor and man's place in nature: A case study in the social construction of neuroanatomy. *Hippocampus* 3:403–415.

Gross, C. G., 1993b. Huxley vs. Owen: The hippocampus minor and evolution. *Trends Neurosci.* 16:493–497.

Gross, C. G., 1994a. Hans-Lukas Teuber: A tribute. *Cereb. Cortex* 5:451–454.

Gross, C. G., 1994b. How inferior temporal cortex became a visual area. *Cereb. Cortex* 5:455–469.

Gross, C. G., 1995. Aristotle on the brain. *Neuroscientist* 1:245–250.

Gross, C. G., 1997a. Emanuel Swedenborg: A neuroscientist before his time. *Neuroscientist* 3:142–147.

Gross, C. G., 1997b. Leonardo da Vinci on the brain and eye. *Neuroscientist,* 3:347–354.

Gross, C. G., 1997c. From Imhotep to Hubel and Wiesel: The story of visual cortex. In: *Cerebral Cortex,* Vol. 13, *Extrastriate Cortex in Primates.* J. H. Kaas, K. Rockland, and A. Peters, eds. Plenum Press, New York.

Gross, C. G., 1998. Galen and the squealing pig. *Neuroscientist,* in press.

Gross, C. G., Bender, D. B., and Gerstein, G. L., 1979. Activity of inferior temporal neurons in behaving monkeys. *Neuropsychology* 17:215–229.

Gross, C. G., Bender, D. B., and Rocha-Miranda, C., 1969. Visual receptive fields of neurons in inferotemporal cortex of the monkey. *Science* 166:1303–1306.

Gross, C. G., and Bornstein, M. H., 1978. Left and right in science and art. *Leonardo* 11:29–38.

Gross, C. G., and Graziano, M. S. A., 1994. Multiple representations of space in the brain. *Neuroscientist* 1:43–50.

Gross C. G., Rocha-Miranda C. E., and Bender D. B., 1972. Visual properties of neurons in inferotemporal cortex of the macaque. *J. Neurophysiol.* 35:96–111.

Gross, C. G., Rodman, H. R., Gochin, P. M., and Colombo, M., 1993. Inferior temporal cortex as a pattern recognition device. In: *Computational Learning and Cognition: Proceedings of the Third NEC Research Symposium.* E. B. Baum, ed. Siam, Philadelphia.

Gross, C. G., Schiller, P. H., Wells, C., and Gerstein, G., 1967. Single-unit activity in temporal association cortex of the monkey. *J. Neurophysiol.* 30:833–843.

Gross, C. G., and Weiskrantz, L., 1964. Some changes in behavior produced by lateral frontal lesions in the macaque. In: *The Frontal Granular Cortex and Behavior.* J. M. Warren, K. Akert, eds. McGraw-Hill, New York.

Gruber, H. E., 1974. *Darwin on Man: A Psychological Study of Scientific Creativity.* Dutton, New York.

Grusser, O. J., and Hagner, M., 1990. On the history of deformation phosphenes and the idea of internal light generated in the eye for the purpose of vision. *Ophthalmology* 74:57–85.

Grusser, O. J., and Landis, T., 1991. Visual agnosias and other disturbances of visual perception and cognition. In: *Vision and Visual Dysfunction.* J. Cronly-Dillon, ed. Macmillan, New York.

Guthrie, D., 1945. *A History of Medicine.* T. Nelson, London.

Harris, S., 1994. *Factories of Death.* Routledge, London.

Hartline, H. K., 1938. The response of single optic nerve fibers of the vertebrate retina. *Am. J. Physiol.* 113:59–60.

Hartline, H. K., and Graham, C. H., 1932. Nerve impulses from single receptors in the eye. *J. Cell. Comp. Physiol.* 1:277–295.

Hécaen, H., and Albert, M. L., 1978. *Human Neuropsychology.* Wiley, New York.

Henschen, S. E., 1893. On the visual path and centre. *Brain* 16:170–180.

Herodotus, 1910. *History,* Vol. I. George Rawlinson, trans. J. M. Dent, London.

Herrlinger, R., 1970. *History of Medical Illustrations from Antiquity to* A.D. 1600. Pitman Medical, London.

Hippocrates, 1950, [4th C. BCE]. On the sacred disease. In: *The Medical Works of Hippocrates.* J. Chadwick, ed. Blackwell, Oxford.

Hofstadter, R., 1955. *Social Darwinism in American Thought.* Beacon, Boston.

Holmes, G. M., 1918a. Disturbance of vision by cerebral lesions. *Br. J. Ophthalmol.* 2:353–384.

Holmes, G. M., 1918b. Disturbances of visual orientation. *Br. J. Ophthalmol.* 2:449–468, 506–516.

Horsley, V. A. H., and Schäfer, E., 1888. A record of experiments upon the functions of the cerebral cortex. *Phil. Trans. R. Soc. Lond.* 179:1–45.

Huang Ti Nei Ching Su Wen, 1949, [4th C. BCE]. *The Yellow Emperor's Classic of Internal Medicine.* I. Veith, trans. Williams & Wilkins, Baltimore.

Hubel, D. H., 1982. Evolution of ideas on the primary visual cortex, 1955–1978: A biased historical account. *Biosci. Rep.* 2:435–469.

Hubel, D. H., 1988. *Eye, Brain and Vision.* Freeman, New York.

Hubel, D. H., and Wiesel, T., 1959. Receptive fields of single neurons in the cat's striate cortex. *J. Physiol.* 148:574–591.

Hubel, D. H., and Wiesel, T., 1962. Receptive fields, binocular interaction and functional architecture in the cat's visual cortex. *J. Physiol.* 160:106–154.

Hubel, D. H., and Wiesel, T., 1965. Receptive fields and functional architecture in two non-striate area visual areas (18 and 19) of the cat. *J. Physiol.* 195:215–243.

Hume, D., 1948. [1739]. An enquiry concerning human understanding. In: *Philosophical Essays Concerning Human Understanding*. L. Selby-Bigge and P. Nidditch, eds. Clarendon, Oxford.

Hunter, R. A., and Macalpine, I., 1963. *Three Hundred Years of Psychiatry, 1535–1860*. Oxford University Press, London.

Hurray, J. B., 1928. *Imhotep: The Vizier and Physician of King Zoser and Afterward the Egyptian God of Medicine*. Oxford University Press, Oxford.

Huxley, L., 1900. *Life and Letters of Thomas Henry Huxley*. Macmillan, London.

Huxley, T. H., 1851. Observations upon the anatomy and physiology of salpa and pyrosoma. *Phil. Trans. Soc. Lond.* 141:567–594.

[Huxley, T. H., 1854]. Review of the *Vestiges of the Natural History of Creation*. *Br. For. Med. Chir. Rev.* 26:425–439.

Huxley, T. H., 1854–1855. Contributions to the anatomy of brachiopoda. *Proc. R. Soc.* 7:241–242.

Huxley, T. H., 1856a. Lectures on general natural history. *Med. Times Gaz.* 12:481–484.

Huxley, T. H., 1856b. Owen and R. Jones on comparative anatomy. *Br. For. Med. Chir. Rev.* 35:325–336.

Huxley, T. H., 1859. On the theory of the vertebrate skull. *Proc. R. Soc.* 9:381–457.

Huxley, T. H., 1861a. On the zoological relations of man with the lower animals. *Nat. Hist. Rev.* 1:67–84.

Huxley, T. H., 1861b. On the brain of *Ateles paniscus*. *Proc. Zool. Soc.* 247–260.

[Huxley, T. H., 1862]. St. Hillaire on the systematic position of man. *Nat. Hist. Rev.* 2:1–8.

Huxley, T. H., 1863. *Evidence as to Man's Place in Nature*. Macmillan, London.

———

Huxley, T. H., 1896. *Man's Place in Nature*. Appelton-Century-Crofts, New York.

Hyvärinen, J., 1982. *The Parietal Cortex of Monkey and Man*. Springer-Verlag, Berlin.

Hyvärinen, J., and Poranen, A., 1974. Function of the parietal associative Area 7 as revealed from cellular discharges in alert monkeys. *Brain* 97:673–692.

Inouye, T., 1909. *Die Sehstörungen bei Schussverletzungen der kortikalen Sehsphäre, nach Beobachtungen an Verwundeten der letzten japanischen Kriege*. W. Englemann, Leipzig.

Irvine, W., 1955. *Apes, Angels and Victorians*. McGraw-Hill, New York.

Iwai, E., and Mishkin, M., 1968. Two visual foci in the temporal lobe of monkeys. In: *Neurophysiological Basis of Learning and Memory*. N. Yoshii and N. Buchwald, eds. Osaka University Press, Osaka.

Jackson, J. H., 1958, [1863–1888]. *Selected Writings of John Hughlings Jackson*. Basic Books, New York.

James, W., 1890. *Principles of Psychology*. Dover, New York.

Jensen, J. V., 1991. *Thomas Henry Huxley: Communicating for Science*. University of Delaware Press, Newark, NJ.

Jonsson, I., 1971. *Emanuel Swedenborg*. Twayne, New York.

Jung, R., 1992. Sensory research in historical perspective: Some philosophical foundations of perception. In: *Handbook of Physiology: The Nervous System*, Vol. III, *Sensory Processes*, Part 1. J. Brookhart and V. Mountcastle, eds. American Physiological Society, Bethesda.

Kaas, J. H., 1997. Theories of extrastriate cortex. In: *Cerebral Cortex*, Vol. 13, *Extrastriate Cortex in Primates*. J. H. Kaas, K. Rockland, and A. Peters, eds. Plenum Press, New York.

Keele, K. D., 1957. *Anatomies of Pain*. Blackwell, Oxford.

Keele, K. D., 1964. Leonardo da Vinci's influence on Renaissance anatomy. *Med. Hist.* 8:360–370.

Keele, K. D., 1977. *Leonardo and the Art of Science.* Wayland, London.

Keith, A., 1925, Huxley as anthropologist. *Nature* 115:697–722.

Kemp, M., 1977. Leonardo and the visual pyramid. *J. Warburg Courtauld Inst.* 40:128–149.

Kemp, M., 1990. *The Science of Art: Optical Themes in Western Art from Brunelleschi to Seurat.* Yale University Press, New Haven, CT.

Kingsley, C., 1863. *Water Babies.* Macmillan, London.

Klüver, H., 1926. Mescal visions and the eidetic types. *Am. J. Psychiatry* 37:502–515.

Klüver, H., 1928. *Mescal, the Divine Plant.* Paul, Trent and Teubner, London.

Klüver, H., 1933. *Behavior Mechanisms in Monkeys.* University of Chicago Press, Chicago.

Klüver, H., 1948. Functional differences between the occipital and temporal lobes with special reference to the interrelations of behavior and extracerebral mechanisms. In: *Cerebral Mechanisms in Behavior.* L. Jeffress, ed. Wiley, New York.

Klüver, H., and Bucy, L., 1938. An analysis of certain effects of bilateral temporal lobectomy in the rhesus monkey, with special reference to "psychic blindness." *J. Psychol.* 5:33–54.

Klüver, H., and Bucy, L., 1939. Preliminary analysis of functions of the temporal lobes in monkeys. *Arch. Neurol. Psychiatry* 42:979–1000.

Konorski, J., 1967. *Integrative Activity of the Brain.* University of Chicago Press, Chicago.

Krieg, W. J. S., 1975. *Interpretive Atlas of the Monkey's Brain.* Brain Books, Evanston, IL.

Kruger, L., 1963. Francois Pourfour du Petit 1664–1741. *Exp. Neurol.* 7:2–5.

Kuffler, S. W., 1953. Discharge patterns and functional organization of mammalian retina. *J. Neurophysiol.* 16:37–68.

Kuypers, H. G. J. M., Szwarcbart, M. K., Mishkin, M., and Rosvold, H. E., 1965. Occipito-temporal cortico-cortical connections in the rhesus monkey. *Exp. Neurol.* 11:245–262.

Lamarck, J. B., 1809. *Philosophie Zoologique.* H. Elliott (1914), trans. *Zoological Philosophy.* Macmillan, London.

Lashley, K. S., 1933. Integrative functions of the cerebral cortex. *Physiol. Rev.* 13:1–42.

Lashley, K. S., 1948. The mechanism of vision. XVIII. Effects of destroying the visual "associative areas" of the monkey. *Genet. Psychol. Monogr.* 37:107–166.

Lashley, K. S., 1950. In search of the engram. *Symp. Exp. Biol.* 4:45–48.

Lashley, K. S., and Clark, G., 1946. The cytoarchitecture of the cerebral cortex of *Ateles:* A critical examination of the architectonic studies. *J. Comp. Neurol.* 85:223–306.

Le Roy Ladurie, E., 1997. *The Beggar and the Professor. A Sixteenth-Century Family Saga,* A. Goldhammer, trans. University of Chicago Press, Chicago.

Lettvin, J. Y., 1995. On grandmother cells, in H. B. Barlow, The neuron doctrine in perception. In: *The Cognitive Neurosciences.* M. S. Gazzaniga, ed. MIT Press, Cambridge.

Lettvin, J. Y., Maturana, H. R., McCulloch, W. S., and Pitts, W. H., 1959. What the frog's eye tells the frog's brain. *Proc. Inst. Radio Engin.* 47:1940–1951.

Lewis, F. T., 1923. The significance of the term hippocampus. *J. Comp. Neurol.* 35:213–230.

Lewy, A., 1847. Ueber die Bedeutung des *Antyllus, Philagrius* und *Posidonius* in der Geschichte der Heilkunde. *Janus* 3:166–184.

Lifton, R. J., 1986. *The Nazi Doctors: Medical Killing and the Psychology of Genocide.* Basic Books, New York.

———

Lindberg, D. C., 1970. The theory of pinhole images from antiquity to the thirteenth century. *Arch. Hist. Exact Sci.* 5:299–325.

Lindberg, D. C., 1976. *Theories of Vision from Al-Kindi to Kepler.* University of Chicago Press, Chicago.

Lissauer, H., 1890. Ein Fall von Seelenblindheit nebst einem Beitrage zur Theorie derselben. *Arch. Psychiatry Nervenkr.* 21:22–270.

Livingstone, M., and Hubel, D., 1988. Segregation of form, color, movement, and depth: Anatomy, physiology, and perception. *Science* 240:740–749.

Lloyd, G. E. R., 1970. *Early Greek Science: Thales to Aristotle.* Norton, New York.

Lloyd, G. E. R., 1973. *Greek Science after Aristotle.* Norton, New York.

Lloyd, G. E. R., 1975. Alcmaeon and the early history of dissection. *Sudhoffs Arch. Geschichte Med.* 59:113–147.

Lloyd, G. E. R., 1978. The Hippocratic question. *Class Q.* 28:202–222.

Locy, W. A., 1911. Anatomical illustration before Vesalius. *J. Morphol.* 22:945–988.

Loeb, J., 1900. *Comparative Physiology of the Brain and Comparative Psychology.* Murray, London.

Lones, T. E., 1912. *Aristotle's Researches in Natural Science.* West Newman, London.

Longrigg, J., 1988. Anatomy in Alexandria in the third century B.C. *Br. J. Hist. Sci.* 21:455–488.

Longrigg, J., 1993. *Greek Rational Medicine: Philosophy and Medicine from Alcmaeon to the Alexandrians.* Routledge, London.

Lyell, C., 1863. *The Antiquity of Man.* Murray, London.

Lynch, J. C., Mountcastle, V. B., Talbot, W. H., and Yin, T. C. T., 1977. Parietal lobe mechanisms for directed visual attention. *J. Neurophysiol.* 40:362–389.

Lyons, J. B., 1966. *The Citizen Surgeon: A Biography of Sir Victor Horsley.* Dawnay, London.

MacCurdy, E., 1954. *The Notebooks of Leonardo da Vinci.* Braziller, New York.

Macko, K. A., Jarvis, C. D., Kennedy, C., Miyaoka, M., Shinohara, M., Sokoloff, L., and Mishkin, M., 1982. Mapping the primate visual system with 2-[^{14}C] deoxyglucose. *Science* 218:394–397.

MacLeod, R. M., 1965. Evolution and Richard Owen. *Isis* 115:259–280.

Malpighi M., 1666. *De cerebri cortice.* Bologna: Montius. Quotation trans. In: *The Human Brain and Spinal Cord.* E. Clarke and C. D. O'Malley (1966), eds. University of California Press, Berkeley.

Manni, E., and Petrosini, L., 1994. Contributions by Bartolomeo Panizza to the anatomy and physiology of some cranial nerves. *J. Hist. Neurosci.* 3:187–197.

Marshall, F. H. A., 1949. Schäfer, Sir Edward Sharpey. In: *Dictionary of National Biography.* L. Stephen and S. Lee, eds. Oxford University Press, London.

Marshall, J., 1861. On the brain of a young chimpanzee. *Nat. Hist. Rev.* 1:296–315.

Martin-Elkins, C. L., and Horel, J. A., 1992. Cortical afferents to behaviorally defined regions of the inferior temporal and parahippocampal gyri as demonstrated by WGA-HRP. *J. Comp. Neurol.* 321:177–192.

Mathe, J., 1980. *Leonardo's Inventions.* D. MacRae, trans. Crescent, New York.

Mayr, E., 1982. *The Growth of Biological Thought.* Harvard University Press, Cambridge.

Mazzarello, P., and Della Sala, S., 1993. The demonstration of the visual area by means of the atrophic degeneration method in the work of Bartolomeo Panizza (1855). *J. Hist. Neurosci.* 2:315–322.

McMurrich, J. P., 1930. *Leonardo da Vinci the Anatomist.* Williams & Wilkins, Baltimore.

Medawar, P. B., and Medawar, J. S., 1983. *From Aristotle to Zoos.* Harvard University Press, Cambridge.

Mesulam, M. M., and Perry, J., 1972. The diagnosis of love-sickness: Experimental psychophysiology without the polygraph. *Psychophysiology* 9:546–551.

Meunier, M., Bachevalier, J., Mishkin, M., and Murray, E. A., 1993. Effects on visual recognition of combined and separate ablations of the entorhinal and perihinal cortex in rhesus monkeys. *J. Neurosci.* 13:5413–5432.

Meyer, A., 1971. *Historical Aspects of Cerebral Anatomy.* Oxford University Press, London.

Meyer, A., and Hierons, R., 1965. On Thomas Willis's concepts of neurophysiology. Part II. *Med. Hist.* 9:142–155.

Milner, A., Ockleford, E. M., and Dewar, W., 1977. Visuo-spatial performance following posterior parietal and lateral frontal lesions in stumptail macaques. *Cortex* 13:350–460.

Minkowski, M., 1911. Zur Physiologie der Sehsphäre. *Pflugers Arch.* 141:171–327.

Mishkin, M., 1954. Visual discrimination performance following partial ablations of the temporal lobe. II. Ventral surface vs. hippocampus. *J. Comp. Physiol. Psychol.* 47:187–193.

Mishkin, M., 1966. Visual mechanisms beyond the striate cortex. In: *Frontiers in Physiological Psychology.* R. W. Russel, ed. Academic Press, New York.

Mishkin, M., and Manning, F. J., 1978. Nonspatial memory after selective prefrontal lesions in monkeys. *Brain Res.* 143:313–323.

Mishkin, M., and Pribram, K., 1954. Visual discrimination performance following partial ablations of the temporal lobe. I. Ventral vs. lateral. *J. Comp. Physiol. Psychol.* 47:14–20.

Mitchell, P. C., 1901. *Thomas Henry Huxley: A Sketch of His Life and Work.* Putnam, New York.

Miyashita, Y., 1993. Inferior temporal cortex: Where visual perception meets memory. *Annu. Rev. Neurosci.* 16:245–263.

Mondino de Luzzi (Mundinus), 1493. *Anothomia.* Romano, Pavia.

Montagu, A., 1959. Introduction to T. H. Huxley, *Man's Place in Nature.* University of Michigan, Ann Arbor, MI.

Morgan, C. L., 1894. *Introduction to Comparative Psychology.* Scott, London.

Morgan, C. T., 1943. *Physiological Psychology.* McGraw-Hill, New York.

Morgan, C. T., and Stellar, E., 1950. *Physiological Psychology,* 2nd ed. McGraw-Hill, New York.

Moore, J., 1979. *The Post-Darwinian Controversies.* Cambridge University Press, Cambridge.

Mountcastle, V. B., 1957. Modality and topographic properties of single neurons of cat's somatic sensory cortex. *J. Neurophysiology* 20:408–434.

Mountcastle, V. B., 1976. The world around us: Neural command functions of selective attention. *Neurosci. Res. Progr. Bull. Suppl.* 14:1–47.

Mountcastle, V. B., Lynch, J. C., Georgopoulos, A., Sakata, H., and Acuna, C., 1975. Posterior parietal association cortex of the monkey: Command functions for operations within extrapersonal space. *J. Neurophysiol.* 38:871–908.

Müller, J. M., 1838. On the specific energies of nerves. In: *A Sourcebook of the History of Psychology.* R. Herrnstein and E. Boring (1965), eds. Harvard University Press, Cambridge.

235

Munk, H., 1881. On the functions of the cortex. In: G. von Bonin (1960), trans. *Some Papers on the Cerebral Cortex.* Charles C Thomas, Springfield, IL.

Nahm, F. K. D., 1997. Heinrich Klüver and the temporal lobe syndrome. *J. His. Neurosci.* 6:193–208.

Needham, J., 1959. *History of Embryology.* Cambridge University Press, Cambridge.

Needham, J., 1983. *Science and Civilization in China,* Vol. 5, *Chemical and Chemical Technology,* Part V. *Spagyrical Discovery and Invention: Physiological Alchemy.* Cambridge University Press, Cambridge.

Nemesius, 1955, [4th C.]. On the nature of man. In: *Cyril of Jerusalem and Nemesius of Emesa.* W. Telfer, ed. Westminster Press, Philadelphia.

Newton, I., 1952, [1704]. *Opticks: Or a Treatise of the Reflections, Refractions, Inflexions, and Colours of Light.* Dover, New York.

Neuburger, M., 1901. Swedenborg's Beziehungen zur Gehirnphysiologie. *Wien. Med. Wochenschr.* 51:2077–2081.

Neuburger, M., 1981 [1897]. *The Historical Development of Experimental Brain and Spinal Cord Physiology Before Flourens.* E. Clarke, trans. Johns Hopkins University Press, Baltimore.

Nordenskiold, E., 1928. *The History of Biology.* Tudor, New York.

Norving, B., and Sourander, P., 1989. Emanuel Swedenborg's theories on the structure and function of the nervous system. In: *Neuroscience Across the Century.* F. C. Rose, ed. Smith-Gordon, London.

Novak, B., 1969. *American Painting of the 19th Century.* Praeger, New York.

Olmstead, E. H., 1967. Historical phases in the influence of Bernard's scientific generalizations in England and America. In: *Claude Bernard and Experimental Medicine.* F. Grande and M. B. Visscher, eds. Schenkman, Cambridge.

O'Malley, C. D., 1964. *Andreas Vesalius of Brussels 1514–1564*. University of California Press, Berkeley.

O'Malley, C. D., and Saunders, J. B., 1952. *Leonardo da Vinci on the Human Body*. Henry Schuman, New York.

Owen, R., 1835. *Descriptive and Illustrative Catalogue of the Physiological Series of the Hunterian Collection*. Taylor, London.

Owen, R., 1848. *The Archetype and Homologies of the Vertebrate Skeleton*. Voorst, London.

Owen, R., 1853. Osteological contributions to the natural history of the chimpanzees and orangs, no. IV. *Trans. Zool. Soc.* 75–88.

Owen, R., 1855. On the anthropoid apes and their relations to man. *Proc. R. Inst.* 2:26–41.

Owen, R., 1858. On the characters, principles of division and primary groups of the class mammalia. *J. Linnaean Soc.* 2:1–37.

Owen, R., 1859. *On the Classification and Geographical Distribution of the Mammalia*. Parker, London.

Owen, R., 1861. On the cerebral characters of man and the ape. *Ann. Mag. Natl. Hist.* 7:456–458.

Owen, R., 1863a. Ape-origin of man as tested by the brain. *Athenaeum,* Feb. 21, 1863.

Owen, R., 1863b. Professor Owen on the human brain. *Athenaeum,* April 11, 1863.

Owen, R., 1866. *On the Anatomy of Vertebrates*. Longmans Green, London.

Owen, R., Rev. 1894. *The Life of Richard Owen*. Murray, London.

Pagel, W., 1958. Medieval and Renaissance contributions to the knowledge of the brain and its functions. In: *The History and Philosophy of Knowledge of the Brain and Its Functions.* F. Poytner, ed. Charles C Thomas, Springfield, IL.

Paget, S., 1949. Horsly, Sir Victor Alexander Holder. In: *Dictionary of National Biography.* L. Stephen and S. Lee, eds. Oxford University Press, London.

Panizza, B., 1855. Osservazioni sul nervo ottico. *G.I. r. lst Lombardo Sci. Lett. Arti. Bibl. Ital.* 7:237–252.

Panofsky, E., 1962. Artist, scientist, genius: notes on the "Renaissance-Dammerung." In: *The Renaissance.* Harper and Row, New York.

Pauly, P. J., 1990. *Controlling Life: Jacques Loeb and the Engineering Ideal in Biology.* University of California Press, Berkeley.

Perrett, D. I., Rolls, E. T., and Caan, W., 1982. Visual neurons responsive to faces in the monkey temporal cortex. *Exp. Brain Res.* 47:329–342.

Plato, 1920, [4th C. BCE]. *The Dialogues of Plato.* B. Jowett, trans. Random House, New York.

Polyak, S. L., 1941. *The Retina.* University Chicago Press, Chicago.

Polyak, S. L., 1957. *The Vertebrate Visual System.* University Chicago Press, Chicago.

Porkert, M., 1974. *The Theoretical Foundations of Chinese Medicine.* MIT Press, Cambridge.

Pribram, K. H., and Bagshaw, M., 1953. Further analysis of the temporal lobe syndrome utilizing fronto-temporal ablations. *J. Comp. Neurol.* 99:347–375.

Rabagliati, A., 1884, 1888. Review of Swedenborg E., 1882, 1887 *The Brain Considered Anatomically, Physiologically and Philosophically.* Speirs, London. *Brain* 6:404–413, and 10:512–524.

———

Ramstrom, M., 1910. *Emanuel Swedenborg's Investigations in Natural Science and the Basis for His Statements Concerning the Functions of the Brain.* University of Uppsala, Uppsala.

Ramstrom, M., 1911. Swedenborg on the cerebral cortex as the seat of psychical activity. In: *Transactions of the International Swedenborg Congress.* Swedenborg Society, London.

Reisch, G., 1503. *Margarita Philosophica.* Schott, Freiburg.

Reti, L., 1974. *The Unknown Leonardo.* McGraw-Hill, New York.

Retzius, G., 1908. The principles of the minute structure of the nervous system as revealed by recent investigations. *Proc. R. Soc. Lond.* 80:414–443.

Richards, E., 1987. A question of property rights: Richard Owen's evolutionism reassessed. *Br. J. Hist. Sci.* 20:85–105.

Richmond, B. J., and Wurtz, R. H., 1982. Inferotemporal cortex in awake monkeys. In: *Changing Concepts of the Nervous System.* A. R. Morrison and P. Strick, eds. Academic Press, New York.

Richter, J. P., 1970. *The Notebooks of Leonardo da Vinci.* Dover, New York.

Ritvo, H., 1987. *The Animal Estate: The English and Other Creatures in the Victorian Age.* Harvard University Press, Cambridge.

Roberts, K. B., and Tomlinson, J. D. W., 1992. *The Fabrics of the Body, European Traditions of Anatomical Illustrations.* Clarendon Press, New York.

Robinson, D. L., Goldberg, M. E., and Stanton, G. B., 1978. Parietal association cortex in the primate: Sensory mechanisms and behavioral modulations. *J. Neurophysiol.* 41:910–936.

Rodman, H. R., 1994. Development of inferior temporal cortex in the monkey. *Cereb. Cortex* 5:484–498.

———

Rolleston, G., 1861. On the affinities of the brain of the orang-utan. *Nat. Hist. Rev.* 1:201–217

Romanes, G. J., 1882. *Animal Intelligence.* Kegan, Paul, and Trench, London.

Ruch, T. C., Fulton, J. F., and German, W. J., 1938. Sensory discrimination in monkey, chimpanzee and man after lesions of the parietal lobe. *Arch. Neurol. Psychiatry* 39:919–938.

Ruderman, D. B., 1995. *Jewish Thought and Scientific Discovery in Early Modern Europe.* Yale University Press, New Haven, CT.

Rupke, N. A., 1994. *Richard Owen: Victorian Naturalist.* Yale University Press, New Haven, CT.

Ruse, M., 1979. *The Darwinian Revolution.* University of Chicago Press, Chicago.

Sarton, G., 1954. *Galen of Pergamon.* University of Kansas Press, Lawrence, KS.

Sarton, G., 1959. *A History of Science,* Vol. 1, *Ancient Science Through the Golden Age of Greece.* Harvard University Press, Cambridge.

Saunders, J. B., and O'Malley, C. D., 1950. *The Illustrations from the Works of Andreas Vesalius of Brussels.* World Publishing Company, Cleveland.

Schäfer, E. A., 1988a. Experiments on special sense localisations in the cortex cerebri of the monkey. *Brain* 10:362–380.

Schäfer, E. A., 1988b. On the functions of the temporal and occipital lobes: A reply to Dr. Ferrier. *Brain* 11:145–161.

Schäfer, E. A., 1900. The cerebral cortex. In: *Textbook of Physiology.* E. Schäfer, ed. Pentland, Edinburgh.

Schiebinger, L., 1993. *Nature's Body.* Beacon Press, Boston.

———

Schiller, F., 1965. The rise of the "enteroid processes" in the 19th century: Some landmarks in cerebral nomenclature. *Bull. Hist. Med.* 41:515–538.

Schiller, F., 1979. *Paul Broca: Founder of French Anthropology, Explorer of the Brain.* University of California Press, Berkeley.

Schlomoh D'Arles, G. B., 1953 [13th C.]. *The Gate of Heaven.* F. S. Bodenheimer, trans. Kiryath Sepher, Jerusalem.

Schneider, G. E., 1967. Contrasting visuomotor functions of tectum and cortex in the golden hamster. *Psychol. Forsch.* 31:52–62.

Schrodinger, E., 1954. *Nature and the Greeks.* Cambridge University Press, Cambridge.

Schroeder van der Kolk, J. L. C., and Vrolik, W., 1849. Nasporingen de Hersenen van den Chimpanzé. In: *Verh. Erste Kl. K. Nederl. Inst. Amsterdam,* 3rd Ser., 1st pt.

Schroeder van der Kolk, J. L. C., and Vrolik, W., 1862. Note sur l'encénphale de l'orang outang. *Nat. Hist. Rev.* 2:111–117.

Secord, J. A., 1989. Behind the Veil: Robert Chambers. In: *History, Humanity, and Evolution: Essays in Honor of John C. Greene.* J. R. Moore, ed. Cambridge University Press, Cambridge.

Sedgwick, A., 1850. *A Discourse on the Studies of the University of Cambridge,* 5th ed., with Additions and a Preliminary Dissertation. Parker, London.

Semmes, J., 1965. A non-tactual factor in astereognosis. *Neuropsychologia* 3:295–315.

Sherrington, C. S., 1935. Sir Edward Sharpey-Schäfer 1850–1935. *Q. J. Exp. Physiol.* 25:99–104.

Siegel, R. E., 1968. *Galen's System of Physiology and Medicine.* S. Karger, New York.

Siegel, R. E., 1970. *Galen on Sense Perception.* S. Karger, New York.

———

Sigerist, H., 1951. *A History of Medicine,* Vol. I, *Primitive and Archaic Medicine.* Oxford University Press, New York.

Sigerist, H., 1961. *A History of Medicine,* Vol. II, *Early Greek, Hindu and Persian Medicine.* Oxford University Press, New York.

Singer, C., 1952. *Vesalius on the Human Brain.* Oxford University Press, London.

Singer, C., 1957. *A Short History of Anatomy and Physiology from the Greeks to Harvey.* Dover, New York.

Skinner, B. F., 1984. *The Shaping of a Behaviorist.* New York University Press, New York.

Smith, H., 1955. *Man and His Gods.* Grosset and Dunlap, New York.

Smith, W. D., 1979. *The Hippocratic Tradition.* Cornell University Press, Ithaca, NY.

Soury, J., 1899. *Le Systeme Nerveux Centrale Structure et Fonctions.* Carre and Naud, Paris.

Spence, J. D., 1985. *The Memory Palace of Matteo Ricci.* Penguin, New York.

Spencer, H., 1855. *Principles of Psychology.* Williams and Norgate, London.

Spillane, J. D., 1981. *The Doctrine of the Nerves, Chapters in the History of Neurology.* Oxford University Press, Oxford.

Spurzheim, J. G., 1834. *Phrenology or the Doctrine of the Mental Phenomenon.* 3rd ed. Marsh, Capen, and Lyon, Boston.

Squires, A. W., 1940. Emanuel Swedenborg and the cerebrospinal fluid. *Ann. Med. Hist.* 2:52–63.

Steckerl, F., 1958. *The Fragments of Praxagoras of Cos and His School.* E. J. Brill, Leiden.

Strong, D. S., 1979. *Leonardo da Vinci on the Eye, an English Translation and Critical Commentary of Ms. D in the Bibliotheque Nationale, Paris, with Studies on Leonardo's Methodology and Theories on Optics.* Garland, New York.

Sur, M., Garraghty, P. E., and Roe, A. W., 1988. Experimentally induced visual projections into auditory thalamus and cortex. *Science* 242:1437–1441.

Suzuki, W. A., and Amaral, D. G., 1994. The perirhinal and parahippocampal cortices of the monkey: Cortical afferents. *J. Comp. Neurol.* 350:3497–3533.

Swedenborg, E., 1843–1844, [1744–1745]. *Regnum animale,* 2 vols. Blyvenburg, The Hague. J. J. G. Wilkinson, trans. *The Animal Kingdom.* Newberry, London.

Swedenborg, E., 1845–1846, [1740–1741]. *Oeconomia regni animalis.* A. Clissold, trans. *The Economy of the Animal Kingdom.* Franc, London.

Swedenborg, E., 1882–1887. *The Brain Considered Anatomically, Physiologically and Philosophically.* R. L. Tafal, trans. Speirs, London.

Swedenborg, E., 1887, [1849]. *De Anima.* Newberry, London. F. Sewall, trans. *The Soul or Rational Psychology.* New Church, New York.

Swedenborg, E., 1914. *The Five Senses.* E. S. Price, trans. Swedenborg Scientific Association, Philadelphia.

Swedenborg, E., 1922. *Psychological Transactions.* A. Acton, trans. Swedenborg Scientific Association, Philadelphia.

Swedenborg, E., 1938. *Three Transactions on the Cerebrum.* A. Acton, trans. Swedenborg Scientific Association, Philadelphia.

Tafel, R L, ed., 1877. *Documents Concerning the Life and Character of Emanuel Swedenborg.* Swedenborg Society, London.

———

Talbot, S. A., and Marshall, W. H., 1941. Physiological studies on neural mechanisms of visual localization and discrimination. *Am. J. Ophthalmol.* 24:1255–1263.

Tamburini, A., 1880. Rivendicazione al Panizza della scoperta del centro visivo cordicale. *Rev. Sper. Frent. Med. Leg.* 6:152–154.

Tanaka, K., 1996. Inferotemporal cortex and object vision. *Annu. Rev. Neurosci.* 19:109–140.

Temkin, O., 1953. Remarks on the neurology of Gall and Spurzheim. In: *Science, Medicine and History,* Vol. II. E. Underwood, ed. Oxford University Press, London.

Teuber, H.-L., 1955. Physiological Psychology. *Annu. Rev. Psychol.* 6:267–296.

Theophrastus, 1917 [4th C. BCE]. On the senses. In: *Theophrastus and the Greek Physiological Psychology Before Aristotle.* G. M. Stratton, trans. Allen and Unwin, London.

Tiedemann, F., 1821. *Icones Cerebri Simiarum et Quorundam Mammalium Rariorum.* Mohr and Winter, Heidelberg.

Tiedemann, F., 1827. Hirn des Orang Outangs mit dem Menschen verglichen, *Z. Allg. Physiol.* 2:17–28.

Tiedemann, F., 1836. On the brain of the Negro compared with that of the European and the orang-outang. *Phil. Trans. R. Soc.* 126:497–527.

Titchener, E. B., 1910. *A Textbook of Psychology.* Macmillan, New York.

Todd, E. M., 1991. *The Neuroanatomy of Leonardo da Vinci.* American Association of Neurology and Surgery, Park Ridge, IL.

Toksvig, S., 1848. *Emanuel Swedenborg.* Yale University Press, New Haven, CT.

Topinard, P., 1878. *Anthropology.* Chapman & Hall, London.

Transactions of the International Swedenborg Congress, 1911. Swedenborg Society, London.

———

Trevarthen, C., 1968. Two mechanisms of vision in primates. *Psychol. Forsch.* 31:299–337.

Ungerleider, L. G., 1995. Functional brain imaging studies of cortical mechanisms for memory. *Science* 270:769–775.

Ungerleider, L. G., and Mishkin, M., 1982. Two cortical visual systems. In: *Analysis of Visual Behavior.* D. Ingle, M. Goodale, and R. Mansfield, eds. MIT Press, Cambridge.

Van Gulik, R. H., 1961. *Sexual Life in Ancient China.* E. J. Brill, Leiden.

Vasari, G., 1987 [1568]. *The Lives of the Artists.* G. Bull, trans. Penguin, London.

Vesalius, A., 1543. *De Humani Corporis Fabrica.* Oporinus, Basel. Quotation trans. In: *The Human Brain and Spinal Cord.* E. Clarke and C. D. O'Malley (1966), eds. University of California Press, Berkeley.

Vicq d'Azyr, F., 1786. *Traite d'Anatomie et Physiologie.* Didot l'Aaine, Paris.

von Bonin, G., and Bailey, P., 1947. *The Neocortex of* Macaca mulatta. University of Illinois Press, Urbana.

von Economo, C., 1929. *The Cytoarchitectonics of the Human Cerebral Cortex.* Oxford University Press, London.

von Helmholtz, H., 1863. *On Sensation of Tone as Physiological Basis for the Theory of Music.* Dover, New York.

von Staden, H., 1989. *Herophilus: The Art of Medicine in Early Alexandria.* Cambridge University Press, Cambridge.

Wallace, A. R., 1891. *Natural Selection and Tropical Nature.* Macmillan, London.

Wallace, A. R., 1905. *My Life: A Record of Events and Opinions.* Chapman & Hall, London.

———

Walshe, F. M., 1958. Some reflections upon the opening phase of the physiology of the cerebral cortex 1850–1900. In: *The History and Philosophy of Knowledge of the Brain and Its Function*. F. Poynter, ed. Charles C Thomas, Springfield, IL.

Ware, J. R., trans., 1966. *Alchemy, Medicine and Religion in the China of 320 A.D; The "Nei Phien" of Ko Hung*. MIT Press, Cambridge.

Webster, M. J., Bachevalier, J., and Ungerleider, L. G., 1994. Connections of inferior temporal areas TEO and TE with parietal and frontal cortex in macaque monkeys. *Cereb. Cortex* 4:470–483.

Wilkinson, J., 1846. *Swedenborg's Economy of the Animal Kingdom*. Walton Mitchell, London.

Wilkinson, J., 1849. *Emanuel Swedenborg: A Biography*. Otis Clapp, Boston.

Willis T., 1684, [1664]. *Cerebri Anatomie*. Martyn and Allestry, London. S. Pordage, trans. as *Dr. Willis's Practice of Physick*. Dring, London.

Wilson, M., 1957. Effects of circumscribed cortical lesions upon somesthetic and visual discrimination in the monkey. *J. Comp. Physiol. Psychol.* 50:630–635.

Wilson, F. A. W., O'Scalaidhe, S. P., and Goldman-Rakic, P. S., 1993. Dissociation of object and spatial processing domains in primate prefrontal cortex. *Science* 260:1955–1958.

Wilson, M., Stamm, J. S., and Pribram, K. H., 1960. Deficits in roughness discrimination after posterior parietal lesions in monkeys. *J. Comp. Physiol. Psychol.* 53:535–539.

Winer, G. A., and Cottrell, J. E., 1996. Does anything leave the eye when we see? Extromission beliefs of children and adults. *Curr. Dir. Psychol. Sci.* 5:137–142.

Witter, M., and Amaral, D. O., 1991. Entorhinal cortex of the monkey: V. Projections to the dentate gyrus, hippocampus and subicular complex. *J. Comp. Neurol.* 307:432–459.

Woolam, D. H. M., 1957. The historical significance of the cerebrospinal fluid. *Med. Hist.* 1:91–114.

Woolam, D. H. M., 1958. Concepts of the brain and its functions in classical antiquity. In: *The History and Philosophy of Knowledge of the Brain and Its Function*. F. Poynter, ed. Charles C Thomas, Springfield, IL.

Woolsey, C. N., 1971. Comparative studies on cortical representation of vision. *Vis. Res. Suppl.* 3:365–382.

Young, R. M., 1970a. The impact of Darwin on conventional thought. In: *The Victorian Crisis of Faith*. A. Symondson, ed. Society for the Promotion of Christian Knowledge, London.

Young, R. M., 1970b. *Mind, Brain and Adaptation in the Nineteenth Century*. Oxford University Press, London.

Young, R. M., 1973. The historiographic and ideological contexts of the nineteenth-century debate on man's place in nature. In: *Changing Perspectives in the History of Science*. M. Teich and R. M. Young, eds. Heinemann, London.

Zimmer, H. R., 1948. *Hindu Medicine*. Johns Hopkins University Press, Baltimore.

Zola-Morgan, S., 1995. Localization of brain function: The legacy of Franz Joseph Gall (1758–1828). *Annu. Rev. Neurosci.* 18:359–383.

Index